The Blending Book

The Blending Book

MAXIMIZING NATURE'S NUTRIENTS

Ann Wigmore
Lee Pattinson

AVERY
a member of Penguin Putnam Inc.

The therapeutic procedures in this book are based on the training, personal experiences, and research of the author. Because each person and situation are unique, the editor and publisher urge the reader to check with a qualified health professional before using any procedure where there is any question as to its appropriateness.

The publisher does not advocate the use of any particular diet or health program, but believes the information presented in this book should be available to the public.

Because there is always some risk involved, the author and publisher are not responsible for any adverse effects or consequences resulting from the use of any of the suggestions, preparations, or procedures in this book. Please do not use the book if you are unwilling to assume the risk. Feel free to consult with a physician or other qualified health professional. It is a sign of wisdom, not cowardice, to seek a second or third opinion.

Front Cover Photo: Envision, NYC
Cover Photographer: Steven Needham
Cover design: Bill Gonzalez
In-house editor: Jennifer L. Santo
Typesetter: Al Berotti

Avery
a member of
Penguin Putnam Inc.
375 Hudson Street
New York, NY 10014
www.penguinputnam.com

Publisher's Cataloging-in-Publication

Wigmore, Ann, 1909-.
    The blending book : maximizing nature's nutrients / Ann Wigmore,
Lee Pattinson.
    p.   cm.
    ISBN: 0-89529-761-2

    1. Blenders (Cookery) 2. Digestive organs—Diseases—Nutritional
aspects. 3. Vegetable juices. 4.Fruit juices.   I. Pattinson,
Lee. II. Title.

TX840.B5W54 1997   641.5′89
                                QBI97-697

Printed in the United States of America

10 9 8 7 6

Contents

This book first is dedicated to my Lord,
who has provided us with ample instruction
on how we should practice nature's law
for an abundant life.

It is also dedicated to all those people
who are affected by so-called "incurable" disorders
who choose not to give up.

And finally, it is dedicated to all those individuals
who are seeking a connection with the source
from which we were created:
God the Father and Earth
the Mother.

Foreword

This book is a fitting climax to Ann Wigmore's life. In her early life Ann experienced poor health. Through her own efforts, she developed a lifestyle that included a nutritional regimen; this lifestyle enabled her to gain health. She presents the nutritional aspect of this regimen in this book, with the hope that it will be adopted by many people for either the attainment or the preservation of their health.

Several years ago, Ann established a clinic in Puerto Rico for the purpose of helping sick people. I went down there for several weeks in 1990 to help in setting up their garden. During this visit, Ann and I had an interesting discussion on longevity. I asked Ann to what age she expected or hoped to live, and she immediately replied that she expected to live to the age of 120, and to retain her good health to the end. When I objected that this was an unreasonable expectation, she countered that there are now many people living to 100 and beyond who have not paid much attention to their diet. How much longer would some of these centenarians live if they had been more diet-conscious in their lifetime? Unfortunately, Ann's life was cut short by an untimely accident, but I believe that she would have reached 120 years, or at least come close. The lesson for the rest of us is that we can not only increase our longevity, but do so in relatively good health, if we adopt a suitable dietary regimen. Life can and should be good, but to enjoy life to the fullest, we must be in good health.

In the approximately twenty-five years I worked with Ann, I would say her promotion of sprouts was her outstanding success. When she started her work, sprouts were almost unheard of, but now they can be regularly found in almost every grocery store and restaurant salad bar. Her most successful innovation was *Rejuvelac,* which is a drink based on sprouts. It is also a key ingredient in many of her dishes. I can endorse *Rejuvelac* wholeheartedly, and I recommend you take what Ann has to say about it to heart.

All of the essentials of Ann's dietary regimen can be found in this book. She tells us what the ideal living foods are, how they are prepared, and how they furnish us with the required nutrients; she also provides detailed explanations of the equipment, procedures, and terminology that are necessary for this regimen. For those who are contemplating this program, as well as for those who have followed it for some time, the recipes are a big help. How did Ann blend these foods into tasty dishes? As she says, once you get the feel for it, you will be able to improvise your own dishes to suit your own tastes.

Some of you who read this book will adopt more of its concepts than others, but regardless of how much you adopt, your health will benefit. Read and enjoy.

— *Harvey Lisle, Ph.D.*

Preface

I was born in Lithuania in 1909. At the age of 16, I came to the United States. I was very anxious to fit into the American Dream. I worked hard in a bakery and made deliveries of bread to factories and homes. When I was 18, both of my legs were broken in a car accident. In the painful days that followed, the doctors discovered that gangrene had set in. I was told that both legs would have to be amputated below the knee. I refused the operation, despite the "death sentence" of my doctors. Remembering how my grandmother used nature for healing, I began to eat everything green I could find. I would lie in the sun and eat the fresh grasses and flowers around me. To the amazement of my family and the doctors, my wounds healed and I completely recovered, with my feet and legs intact.

Later in life, after drifting back to more ordinary ways of eating, I began to suffer from arthritis, migraine headaches, and colon cancer. At age fifty, I had gray hair and felt like an old woman. It was at this point that I decided to change my lifestyle. Once again, I began to eat only uncooked foods, such as fresh fruits and vegetables, along with freshly gathered weeds and grasses. At the same time, I began experimenting with growing wheatgrass and indoor greens. Later, I developed sprouting methods for seeds and grains. My digestive system could not handle even sprouted seeds, so I developed techniques for fermentation, for juicing fresh, chlorophyll-rich wheatgrass, and for blending food for easy-to-digest nourishment. My health problems completely reversed themselves. My hair returned to its natural color, and my energy level allowed me to work eighteen to twenty hours a day!

This "living foods" program was so successful for me that I began to teach it to other persons who could not be helped with drugs. The results were equally amazing. Their aches and discomforts disappeared and their skepticism turned to anticipation at being able to enjoy good health again.

After being saved from the grip of disease and death, I believe that health is our birthright when we follow nature's simple laws. The body will heal itself of any illness when it is given living, enzyme-rich, easy-to-digest nourishment. Anyone can experience the benefits of such nourishment in just two to four weeks of blended living foods. I believe we can have a world without disease and suffering, if we are willing to turn back to nature, and I have written *The Blending Book* to show how this can be done.

In *The Blending Book*, I examine how the modern diet puts a tremendous burden on our digestive systems and leads to numerous health problems. I then explain how blending living foods can correct these problems by providing us with maximum nutrients for less internal effort; with less stress on the digestive system, the body will be able to heal itself. I also provide detailed information about the valuable nutrients contained in living foods, instructions on blending equipment and techniques, and delicious, kitchen-tested blending recipes.

Through the simple act of blending, you can restore or maintain optimum health. In *The Blending Book*, you will find all the information you need to get started.

1

What Is the Living Foods Lifestyle?

The living foods lifestyle is more than just a diet; it is a way of taking total responsibility for your nutritional needs. Living foods are the most nutritious foods that exist, and they are all offered in an easy-to-digest form. Living foods include super-nutritious young organic greens; power-packed sprouted nuts, seeds, and grains; and fabulous fermented preparations. In addition, fresh wheatgrass juice adds an unparalleled level of nutritional healing and vitality. All of these foods are prepared without cooking, since cooking destroys the life force in the enzymes. The living foods lifestyle uses no meat, dairy foods, or other animal products. As you will learn, there is no need for these most destructive foods; living foods provide all the nutrients your body needs.

Before we go into a thorough discussion of living foods, I would like to clarify some important points that have been a source of much confusion. First of all, living foods are not the same as raw foods. Because of the unprecedented severe digestion and assimilation

problems that now exist, the average person cannot digest raw foods. Even a simple sprout salad can present
major digestive problems for most people. Foods such
as hard root vegetables, tough fibrous vegetables, and
unsprouted nuts, seeds, and grains are indigestible. The
living foods lifestyle incorporates these foods through
special preparation techniques such as sprouting, fermentation, and blending with *Rejuvelac* (a drink made
from sprouted wheatberries) for easy digestion.

Those new to the living foods lifestyle may be in-
clined to think they have joined the vanguard of a
brand-new era in the world of eating and nutrition.
They may feel as though they are pioneers, and are, as
the well-known saying has it, "boldly going where no
man has gone before." The truth is that we at the Ann
Wigmore Foundation have simply turned back the clock,
as it were, and are following a way of life that was
part of the day-to-day experience of those who lived
many, many years ago.

But some may protest, "Surely blending, which is
a very important part of the living foods lifestyle, is
something new." If blending makes you think only of
an electric blender, mixing food with incredible speed
and thoroughness, well, yes, that is a product of comparatively recent times. But "blending," or combining
different ingredients to make food more digestible, has
been with us since long before electricity was invented,
or even imagined.

THE EARLIEST ORIGINS OF BLENDING

Caves have been found all over the world whose walls
are covered with ancient drawings. These drawings may
be crudely executed, but they still clearly record the
daily lifestyle of the people who drew them.

In these drawings, it is not unusual to see a figure with a bowl in front of it and a short, thick stick in its hand. Or there may be a drawing of a figure leaning over a rock placed on top of another rock; even from the sparse lines of the sketch, one can see that something is being pressed between the two surfaces. These figures are pounding grain in bowls or crushing it between two stones, sometimes mixing the end result with water, honey, or another additive. In other words, they are blending their food to make it more palatable—easier to eat and digest—exactly as we do today.

VEGETABLES: THE ANCIENT STAPLE

Our ancient ancestors always included raw vegetables as a staple in their diets. Those who settled in a particular area and developed territorial rights grew them purposefully. Those who remained nomadic sought them out on the trail.

Dwindling numbers of modern-day primitive cultures throughout the world still incorporate raw vegetables as a dietary staple. In Australia, for instance, there are still some nomadic aborigines who live "off the bush" on berries, leaves, and wild fruits. In addition, some areas of Africa and South America, such as the Amazon basin, still contain small groups who derive most of their sustenance from what grows naturally, and not from cultivated gardens or fields.

Even the earlier-civilized countries have long eaten foods that are only now being slowly integrated into the Western diet. For example, small, red, sweet-flavored adzuki beans originated in China, where their nutritional value—they contain iron to stave off anemia, immunity-raising zinc, and B complex vitamins to aid immune system function—has made them part of the Chinese diet for many generations.

China also introduced us to chow-chow, a combination of fresh garden vegetables. Chinese laborers working on the American railroads in the nineteenth century brought this familiar delicacy with them to their new land. Chow-chow is cholesterol-free and high in vitamin C, iron, and potassium. Because it is pickled, its sodium content is higher than is now thought desirable. This is not considered a problem for the Chinese, however, because they eat it in very moderate amounts and usually combine it with a very healthy diet.

LIVING FOODS IN THE BIBLE

The Bible is full of references to the very types of foods that we use in the living foods lifestyle. Onions, cucumbers, melons, leeks, and garlic were all familiar at that time. Fresh and dried figs, grapes, raisins, and pomegranates are mentioned, as well as different kinds of nuts, especially almonds and pistachio nuts. Grain, of course, was a staple, and it was always soaked before being baked into bread. Today we know that this removes the enzyme inhibitors and allows us to get more of the life force from the grain.

Honey was widely used, mainly as a sweetener. Samson found honey in the carcass of a lion; Jonathan found it in the forest; and Moses found it in a rock. Jacob sent honey to Joseph in Egypt, and there is a mention of it being exported to the Phoenicians. Honey can be used in small quantities in many of these recipes when a little sweetness is wanted.

AMARANTH AND THE AZTECS

Amaranth seeds mixed with honey were used as a food by the ancient Aztecs, though it is unlikely that they had any idea of its high nutritional value. As is often seen in the recordings of ancient civilizations, there seems to have been an instinct for what was healthy or curative, even if there was no way of knowing just why it was so.

Amaranth has tiny green flowers growing in dense clusters. The plant grows wild along roadsides in the United States, especially in the late summer and fall. Although it was long regarded here only as a weed, in Europe it can be found as a cultivated garden plant. But today Americans are beginning to recognize its value, and it can now be found in health food stores. In addition to the seeds, the young leaves can be added to salads. Amaranth is packed full of vitamins, especially A, C, E, and some B complex vitamins. It also contains twice the protein of other leafy vegetables.

People today continue to blend food when it is necessary or appropriate—for example, for babies with no teeth and immature digestive systems, or for elderly people who have lost their teeth, and who, as a result, cannot digest food unless it is blended. As you can see, the foods used in the living foods lifestyle are far from being new, though their return to popularity may have been fairly recent. In many cases, this is the result of findings in our modern laboratories, where scientists are now slowly uncovering nutrition "secrets" that were once known to everyone.

2

Why Blend?

Perhaps the question most frequently asked by those beginning to practice the living foods lifestyle is, "Why blend practically everything that is eaten?" The answer is simple. Blending is the easiest and most efficient way to provide food that is both nourishing and easy to digest. By blending foods, we can counteract the poor eating habits most of us have developed over the years, and that are the cause of many of the physical problems we have.

It has long been known that what we eat directly affects our health. The average American diet consists mainly of processed junk foods that are high in fat, cholesterol, salt, and sugar, and low in fresh fruits and vegetables and whole grains. Eventually, this type of intake leads to digestive troubles, obesity, heart disease, and cancer, as well as nutrient deficiencies that cause a host of problems of their own.

However, a diet that is rich in fresh vegetables and fruits, whole grains, sprouts, seeds, and nuts contains the nutrients we need to fight off these and other diseases. If we go a step further and blend these foods, we can be certain that we will receive their full nutritional benefit. When food is cooked or otherwise processed, valuable nutrients are destroyed, but this is not the case with blending. It insures that the food we eat is suitably prepared for absorption and assimilation into the body, with all nutrients intact.

BLENDING FOR BETTER HEALTH

Blending is equally appropriate for people who are ill and people who are healthy. If you are ill, blending your food will relieve your body of some of the extra effort required for digestion, so this energy may be better spent on healing.

Because of the severe digestive problems so many people face, in addition to other illnesses, it is imperative to have a means to help the body assimilate nourishment. Blending is a wonderful solution to this problem, because it is an easy way to provide a complete meal containing all the nutrients you need to fight off your illness. Blending living foods with *Rejuvelac*, for example, prevents the loss of vitamins because the vitamin E in the *Rejuvelac* acts as an antioxidant. Adding shredded carrot, zucchini, or other vegetables to your blended mixtures will provide extra fiber, which is very important for digestive health.

If you are healthy, blending will help you to stay that way. Blended living foods are full of vitamins, minerals, enzymes, and other nutrients, and since they are easy to digest and assimilate, they give your body more of what it needs to keep functioning at top condition. The most important key to health is to use blended foods in small amounts frequently throughout the day. I realize that this may seem drastic, but if you are serious about maintaining or restoring your health, I can assure you that this is the most beneficial way. And remember, the living foods lifestyle is a guide for the highest level of health, in which the body is free of illness and full of energy.

I have seen so many students come to my centers with all kinds of diseases. There is absolutely no doubt in my mind that every one of these people suffers from an inability to assimilate nourishment, which leads to deficiencies and illness. When easy-to-digest, high-energy blended foods are provided, the changes in their health are immediate. Unfortunately, in our society, unhealthy eating habits, and therefore illnesses, tend to prevail.

OUR SOCIETY'S EATING PROBLEM

In our society, we tend to eat food in chunks, swallowing it quickly after very little chewing. This means that the enzymes in the mouth do not have a chance to start the digestive process by breaking down the starch content of our food. As a result, as the food progresses through the digestive tract, it is inadequately prepared for assimilation. This, in turn, means that much of the nutrition the food should provide is not absorbed, and is eventually excreted as waste.

Years of poor eating habits are likely to have an adverse effect on the entire system by physiologically altering its structure; a person with a poor digestive system will not have a healthy, balanced body. A domestic equivalent can be seen in any household plumbing system. Bombard it for years with waste, without taking any steps to maintain or clean it, and eventually the pipes will clog. The same applies to the body's "pipes." One of the reasons that I include enemas and high-colonic therapy in my suggested regimen is to give the

body an opportunity to restore the optimum conditions
needed for total assimilation of all nutrients.

Another common habit in our society is eating
three times a day, at regular intervals, whether we are
hungry or not. A clock-ruled schedule is not the answer
to digestive problems. We should eat only when we are
hungry, and *never* when we are stressed or angry. Eating quickly causes blood to rush to the digestive tract
in order to cope with the demand, and this is done at
the expense of the rest of the body.

One practice I encourage—and follow myself when-
ever possible—is that of taking individual meals on
trays, instead of with a group at a table. An alternative
is to have one of the day's meals designated as a "silent
meal." Unfortunately, it is common for people to use
any gathering as a forum for airing problems or griev-
ances, aches and pains, and the troubles of the world
in general, with most of the conversation being negative
in content. This is hardly conducive to tranquil meal-
times, and very likely to produce some degree of stress.

For many people, a short fast will be beneficial to
their health. This period should never last more than
one to three days, but it will give the digestive tract a
chance to relax and will improve enzymatic function. As
Gabriel Cousens, M.D., explains: "During a fast, the natural bacteria in our bodies have the opportunity to add
a great deal of their enzymes to our system, and so increase our total enzyme force. When fasting, the body
stops producing digestive enzymes and the enzyme energy is diverted to the metabolic sphere of operation,
which includes an increased rate of breakdown of the
old cells as well as an elimination of fatty deposits, in-
complete proteins, and other toxic materials in the system. The enzymes become a rejuvenating power for us."

We all have known people who, though they eat
enormous amounts of food, remain undernourished and

are never completely healthy. This is because their digestive systems are faulty, and they do not benefit from the nutrition in the food they eat. An unhealthy diet leads to a digestive system that can't function properly. Living foods have been developed so that even the most severe digestive problems can be overcome through easy-to-digest, high-energy nourishment. Every food allows your body to receive optimal nutrition.

Blending the right types of food means that the body will have a chance to recover from those years of abuse or neglect, and, while it recovers, it will be relieved of the extra effort required to digest and absorb its intake. Blended foods are easy to digest and assimilate, but solid foods, such as easy-to-chew uncooked vegetables, cannot be avoided, because the body needs a certain amount of fiber for elimination. My personal opinion is that a diet should consist of 70 percent blended foods and 30 percent other living foods. But each person has a different system and different needs; one must learn to listen to his or her own body.

HOW THE DIGESTIVE SYSTEM WORKS

I must confess that I took it somewhat for granted that everyone knows just how the human digestive system works. It was not until I began asking around that I realized how many misconceptions there are about this very important system. Even people whom I had assumed would have at least a working knowledge of the digestive process were alarmingly misinformed or undereducated.

The digestive system is not simply a tube, open at both ends, with permeable walls through which food is assimilated. Instead, it is the site of an extremely complex and orderly process involving the mechanical and chemical breakdown of food in designated stages. This combination of mechanical and chemical action alters the structure of the food. Any food that remains, unabsorbed and unused, passes through the large intestine and is excreted as waste.

An outline of the process of digestion will make it easier to understand both how our systems have been damaged by modern eating habits, and how blending can help correct this damage easily and effectively.

The Mouth

The physical breakdown of food begins in the mouth when we chew. The chemical breakdown of food is started by the salivary glands and enzymes present in the mouth. The organs of smell as well as taste help stimulate the three salivary glands—this is how the phrase "mouth-watering smell" originated. The salivary glands secrete mucus and a digestive enzyme called salivary amylase. The mucus moistens the food and allows it to pass easily through the esophagus (the tube that runs from the mouth to the stomach). The salivary amylase begins the chemical digestion of carbohydrates. Failure to thoroughly chew your food renders this phase ineffective and makes the work of other sections of the digestive system more difficult. Blending your food makes up for this failure.

The Esophagus

The esophagus is a tube, approximately ten inches long in adults, that provides a passageway from the mouth to the stomach. However, it plays no part in the actual digestion of food. Its lining is designed to resist abrasion by any large or coarse items of food that may pass through it.

At the lower end of the esophagus is a muscle called the cardiac sphincter. Once food passes through the cardiac sphincter into the stomach, the main digestion process begins.

The Stomach

The stomach is lined with a mucus membrane that contains thousands of microscopic gastric glands. These glands secrete hydrochloric acid and various enzymes. The muscular walls of the stomach contract to mix the food thoroughly with the hydrochloric acid and enzymes, producing a naturally blended, smooth substance called chyme.

Protein digestion starts in the stomach, where two enzymes in the gastric juices—rennin and pepsin—break up the very large protein molecules into simpler compounds. Other enzymes—trypsin in the pancreatic juice and peptidases in the intestinal juices—continue the protein digestion later on. Every protein molecule consists of many amino acids; when these molecules are split up into separate amino acids by the enzymes, protein digestion is complete.

Food is held in the stomach cavity by the pyloric sphincter muscle until this partial digestion is finished. This takes an average of three hours for most foods. The chyme then passes through the pyloric sphincter into the small intestine.

The Small Intestine

Like the mucus lining of the stomach, that of the small intestine also has thousands of microscopic glands that secrete digestive juices. The small intestine's multifolded structure, called a *plica*, is covered by thousands of tiny "fingers" called *villi*. Each of the villi contains a rich network of capillaries to absorb the sugars and amino acids that are the products of carbohydrate and protein digestion. Since the plica is folded, it has a very large surface area that allows rapid absorption of food into the blood and lymphatic systems. Each villus contains a lymphatic vessel, called a *lacteal gland,* that absorbs lipids or fat materials from the chyme. The villus itself is covered by cells with a border called *microvilli,* that further increase the surface area for the absorption of nutrients.

The small intestine is made up of three sections: the duodenum, the jejunum, and the ileum. Most chemical digestion occurs in the duodenum, or first section. Chyme from the stomach, which is acidic in nature, passes into this area, where a comparatively modern problem—the duodenal ulcer—sometimes occurs. It is generally accepted that prolonged hyperacidity is one of the main causes of ulcers, along with stress and other emotional states such as anxiety, and the hasty swallowing of insufficiently chewed meals. Blending of foods can overcome this problem.

Pancreatic digestive juices and bile—made in the liver and stored in the gallbladder—empty into the middle third of the duodenum through ducts. Another comparatively modern problem that occurs here is jaundice, which is the result of the blocking of one or more of these ducts. This is often due to the inability to properly digest food, so blending can help this problem by providing food that is already partially digested.

The Liver, the Gallbladder, and the Pancreas

Most people do not fully appreciate the importance of the liver, the gallbladder, and the pancreas in the digestive process.

The liver produces bile, which is then stored in the gallbladder. Because fats form in large globules, they must be broken down into small particles for absorption. This is the function of bile. Fats in the chyme trigger secretions of the hormone cholecystokinin, which, in turn, stimulates the contraction of the gallbladder to start the flow of the bile. This hormone also stimulates the release of enzymes from the pancreas.

In addition to the production of bile, the liver cells have other important functions. They play a major role in the metabolism of all kinds of food, help maintain normal blood glucose concentration, start the first steps of protein and fat metabolism, and synthesize several kinds of protein compounds. Liver cells can also help detoxify various substances, such as bacterial products and certain drugs. They also store iron and vitamins A, B_{12}, and D.

Pancreatic juice is also a very important digestive aid. It contains enzymes that digest all three major kinds of food—protein, fat, and starch. It also contains sodium bicarbonate, an alkaline substance that neutralizes the hydrochloric acid in the gastric juices. In addition, the pancreas houses the islets of Langerhans, which are cells that make insulin.

Very little digestion of carbohydrates occurs in the mouth or stomach because, as mentioned earlier, most of us swallow our food so fast that the salivary amylase usually has little time to do its work, and gastric juice contains no carbohydrate-digesting enzymes. It is when the food reaches the small intestine that pancreatic and intestinal juices digest these starches and sugars.

The process begins when the enzyme, pancreatic amylase, changes starches into a sugar, maltose. Then the three intestinal enzymes—maltase, sucrase, and lactase—digest the sugars by changing them into simple sugars, mainly glucose (or dextrose). Maltase digests maltose (malt sugar), sucrase digests sucrose (ordinary cane sugar), and lactase digests lactose (milk sugar).

Digestion of fat also does not occur before the small intestine is reached, and again, the pancreas is involved in this process. Gastric lipase, an enzyme in the gastric juice, does digest some fat in the stomach, but most goes undigested until the bile in the small intestine breaks down the large fat globules. Then a pancreatic enzyme, steapsin or pancreatic lipase, splits the molecules into fatty acids and glycerol.

The Large Intestine

In the large intestine, any material that has escaped digestion in the small intestine is acted upon by bacteria, so additional nutrients may be released here from cellulose and other fibers. The bacteria in this section are responsible for the synthesis of vitamin K—needed for normal blood clotting and liver function—and for the production of some of the B complex vitamins that, once formed, are absorbed into the bloodstream. Anything that is not absorbed here is excreted as waste, and again, blending is useful for this purpose, since it provides nourishment that is more easily and completely absorbed.

METABOLISM

Metabolism is the use the body makes of what has been eaten, digested, absorbed, and channeled to the cells.

Food is used in one of two ways—as a source of energy or as building blocks for making complex chemical compounds that enable the body to function in a variety of ways. The food must be processed and absorbed into the cells, then undergo many changes, before either of these things can occur.

The chemical reactions that release energy from food molecules make up the process of catabolism; this is the only way the body has of supplying itself with the energy needed to perform many different functions. The process of building food molecules into complex chemical compounds is called anabolism.

Together, catabolism and anabolism make up the process called metabolism. The Basal Metabolic Rate (BMR) is the number of calories of heat that must be available each day, simply to keep an individual alive and functioning. Additional nutrition is necessary to enable him or her to have energy for working and other activities. The more active a person is, the more food he or she must metabolize.

This in itself is the best argument for blending foods—blending enables the body to utilize its energy to the maximum by making all the nutrients easily absorbable and digestible, with minimum effort on the part of the system.

Once we eliminate foods that affect us adversely from our diet, and become accustomed to foods of high nutritional value, we will be a long way down the road to ridding ourselves of many health problems that have plagued us, and that we may have accepted as "part of life."

As the body regains its health, it will once again produce its own enzymes and be free of digestive problems, and intake can gradually embrace a wider range of foods. Until this happens, there can be little question that the blending proposed in my regimen is the answer to those troublesome assimilation and digestive problems, and will insure they do not recur.

3

The Nutrients We Need and Where to Find Them

As I discussed in the previous chapter, when we fail to chew our food thoroughly, the entire digestive system must work even harder to insure that we digest and absorb all the nutrients we need. If, in addition to these poor eating habits, the food itself is low in nutrients, many health problems can result. These problems can be solved by blending our food for easier digestion and assimilation, and by making sure that what we eat is rich in the nutrients we need for good health.

But what are these nutrients, and how can we obtain them from our diet? This chapter will provide a brief overview of the necessary nutrients, and the foods that contain them. The charts at the end of the book will provide additional information.

NUTRITION AND THE IMMUNE SYSTEM

The immune system can best be described as the body's

protector. Its task is to identify, track, and destroy the body's potential enemies before they can do any major harm.

Any protector, to do the job properly, must always be at the peak of condition, so it is absolutely essential that your body gets the nutrition it needs to stay constantly at that "battle-ready" peak. What you eat—and how well it is digested and absorbed—can either strengthen or weaken your immune system. Your intake provides the elements necessary for building and maintaining the millions of cells the immune system needs to do its job. If there is a deficiency of any of these elements, the immune system—and the rest of the body—cannot function properly. This is why blending is so effective—it allows more nutrients to be absorbed into the body from your food. In addition, the foods you blend are naturally high in nutrients.

I cannot emphasize enough the importance of blended foods in order to give the body a chance to assimilate nourishment to supply the missing elements. Energy Soup (see page 73), for example, is a complete meal, containing every nutrient that the body needs in a balanced form.

We need vitamins to strengthen the immune system. For example, it has long been known that a deficiency of vitamin C weakens this system, and that the B complex vitamins are essential for producing germ-fighting antibodies. Minerals, especially zinc and selenium, also have a profound effect on the immune system. However, an excess of some minerals (such as copper, cadmium, and lead) can reduce the body's fighting abilities.

Vitamins and minerals are not the only nutrients the immune system needs to stay in top condition. Amino acids, enzymes, and chlorophyll are not as well-known, but are equally important. For example, many people who suffer from allergic conditions have a deficiency of enzymes, and as a result, their immune systems have been weakened. They have problems assimilating food, and often problems with elimination, as well. All these can be aided by an initial blending of foods to make a complete and nourishing meal.

VITAMINS

Vitamins are needed for normal growth, tissue maintenance, and metabolism. They also work with enzymes to insure that all the body's activities are carried out properly. Vitamins and minerals are called *micronutrients* because they are only needed in small amounts. Because most are not made by the body, they must be obtained from the diet. As with other nutrients, a deficiency of just one vitamin can cause problems for the entire body.

There is no substitute for the vitamins obtained from live foods. Like enzymes, many vitamins are destroyed in the cooking process, but this does not occur when foods are blended. In addition, vitamins in live foods are often naturally combined with other nutrients for maximum absorption and use by the body; this is not something that can be duplicated in vitamin pills.

The following list should give you an idea of which vitamins can be found in various living foods. For more information, consult the charts at the back of this book.

- *Vitamin A:* This can be found in alfalfa, apricots, asparagus, beet greens, broccoli, cantaloupe, carrots, collards, dandelion greens, dulse, garlic, kale, kelp, mustard greens, papayas, peaches, pumpkins, red peppers, spinach, sweet potatoes, Swiss chard, turnip greens, watercress, and yellow squash.

- *Vitamin B₁ (thiamine):* Legumes, peas, and whole grains are the best sources, but this is also found in alfalfa, asparagus, broccoli, Brussels sprouts, dulse, kelp, nuts, plums, prunes, raisins, and watercress.

- *Vitamin B$_2$ (riboflavin):* The best sources are legumes, spinach, and whole grains. Vitamin B$_2$ is also found in alfalfa, asparagus, avocados, broccoli, Brussels sprouts, currants, dandelion greens, dulse, kelp, leafy green vegetables, mushrooms, nuts, and watercress.

- *Vitamin B$_3$ (niacin):* This is found in alfalfa, broccoli, carrots, dandelion greens, dates, potatoes, and tomatoes.

- *Vitamin B$_5$ (pantothenic acid):* This is found in fresh vegetables, legumes, mushrooms, and nuts.

- *Vitamin B$_6$ (pyroxidine):* All foods contain some vitamin B$_6$, but those with the highest concentration are carrots, peas, spinach, and sunflower seeds.

- *Vitamin B$_{12}$ (cyanocobalamin):* This is not found in many vegetables, except sea vegetables (such as dulse, kelp, kombu, and nori), soybeans and soy products, and alfalfa.

- *Biotin (B complex vitamin):* This is found in soybeans and whole grains.

- *Choline:* This is found in legumes, soybeans, and whole grain cereals.

- *Folic acid:* This is found in dates, green leafy vegetables, legumes, lentils, mushrooms, oranges, root vegetables, and whole grains.

- *Inositol:* This is found in fruits, legumes, raisins, vegetables, and whole grains.

- *PABA:* This is found in mushrooms, spinach, and whole grains.

- *Vitamin C (ascorbic acid):* This is found in berries, citrus fruits, and green vegetables.

- *Vitamin D:* This is found in dark greens, sweet potatoes, alfalfa, and parsley.

- *Vitamin E:* This is found in dark green leafy vegetables, legumes, nuts, seeds, and whole grains.

- *Vitamin K:* This is found in alfalfa, asparagus, broccoli, Brussels sprouts, cabbage, cauliflower, dark green leafy vegetables, kelp, and soybeans.

MINERALS

The body requires minerals for the composition of body fluids, the building of blood and bones, healthy nerve function, and muscle tone. The chemical balance of the body depends on the levels of minerals in the body. If one level is out of balance, all the others are affected; this can cause other imbalances, and lead to illness.

As is the case with vitamins and other nutrients, minerals do not stand up well to cooking. The minerals found in live foods are chelated—that is, bound to amino acids for easier assimilation. When foods are cooked, these bonds are broken, and the minerals are not absorbed as easily. Blending, however, does not affect these bonds. Although chelated minerals are available in supplement form, it is still better to obtain them from live foods, because the combinations that occur in nature cannot be duplicated in the laboratory.

The following list should give you an idea of what minerals can be found in living foods. For more information, consult the charts at the back of this book.

- *Calcium:* This is found in green leafy vegetables, dulse, kelp, figs, prunes, tofu, and alfalfa.

- *Iodine:* This is found in sea vegetables, such as kelp, dulse, and others.

- *Iron:* This is found in green leafy vegetables, whole grains, dates, dulse, kelp, peaches, pears, prunes, pumpkins, raisins, soybeans, watercress, and alfalfa.

- *Potassium:* This is found in apricots, avocado, bananas, dates, dulse, figs, dried fruit, garlic, potatoes, nuts, raisins, winter squash, and yams.

- *Zinc:* This is found in dulse, kelp, legumes, mushrooms, pumpkin seeds, soybeans, sunflower seeds, whole grains, and alfalfa.

THE IMPORTANCE OF ENZYMES

Enzymes are protein compounds that we need to survive. They are involved in nearly every activity that takes place within our bodies, including digestion. Unfortunately, many scientists fail to realize just how necessary enzymes are to human life, and as a result, the importance of including enzymes in our diet is often overlooked.

Enzymes are fragile substances. Cooking food at temperatures higher than 118°F destroys its natural enzymes, as well as many of the vitamins needed for optimum health. Caffeine is an enemy to enzymes, as are strong spices and vinegar. This means that the caffeine content of the coffee, tea, and cola drinks we often take with our meals effectively blocks the natural process of digestion from the beginning. Even cold drinks and such things as sugar, salt, and bleached flour inhibit enzyme function. This is one of the best reasons why blending and a living foods lifestyle are ideal; live foods are full of enzymes, and blending, unlike cooking, leaves the enzymes and other nutrients intact.

Enzymes are divided into two main groups: metabolic and digestive. Metabolic enzymes act as catalysts, promoting or speeding up the numerous chemical reactions in the body. They are also responsible for the building and repairing of cells, among other functions. Digestive enzymes are present in the digestive tract, and are responsible for breaking down food.

Humans are born with a certain amount of enzymes; we can also get them from food. Enzymes obtained this way help to digest what we eat. If we don't get enough enzymes from our food, we must draw on our supply of metabolic enzymes to aid in digestion. This means there are fewer enzymes available for other functions in the body, such as cleansing and repair. This enzyme imbalance eventually leads to illnesses, including allergies, obesity, heart disease, and some forms of cancer.

By blending fresh, raw, organically grown foods, we not only relieve our metabolic enzymes of the extra job of digestion, but we add to the store of enzymes in our body. Another advantage of blending is that a very satisfying meal can be obtained from a relatively small amount of food. This further relieves the enzymes in the digestive tract and avoids the overworking of a long-overburdened system.

THE IMPORTANCE OF AMINO ACIDS

Our knowledge of the functioning and values of amino acids is still in its infancy, though in recent years a great deal has been learned. It seems clear, however, that amino acids are of immense importance to our overall health.

It is known that amino acids are a combination of various elements—carbon, hydrogen, oxygen, and in some cases, sulfur—and that they are the raw materials needed by the body to make many of its necessary compounds, such as enzymes, neurotransmitters, and some forms of saccharides. They are also important for proper digestion and assimilation, cell renewal, rapid healing, and immunity.

Amino acids are divided into two groups—essential and nonessential. This does not mean that one type is more important than the other; essential amino acids are those that we must get from our diet, because the body cannot manufacture them. A deficiency of just one amino acid can cause numerous health problems. Sprouts and leafy green vegetables are the best sources of amino acids, and blending is an excellent way to obtain them in an easy-to-digest form.

Amino acid therapy has been shown to be valuable in treating certain conditions, such as some forms of depression and herpes infections, some weight problems involving the metabolic system, insomnia, and epilepsy. There also seems to be little doubt that the concentration of amino acids and a B complex vitamin called choline in the blood has a definite bearing on the ability of the neurons in the brain to manufacture and use their transmitters.

Individual requirements for amino acids vary enormously, depending on so many factors—height, weight, age, energy level needed, genetic influences, stresses such as illnesses or infections, and natural conditions such as pregnancy—that it is really impossible at this stage to determine even an average level of need until more is known. It seems certain that amino acids will be increasingly used and accepted as a new therapeutic tool with which to treat many conditions, and as our overall knowledge of them increases, so, too, will our application of them.

CHLOROPHYLL

It has recently been recognized that chlorophyll, a natural element in plants, is much more important to our health than was previously thought. Chlorophyll is created in plants as a result of a conversion of the sun's energy; when we eat plants containing chlorophyll, this vital energy is transferred to us. In addition, the chlorophyll molecule is very similar to that of hemoglobin, which carries oxygen in the blood. Many experiments have shown that animals can enrich their blood by converting chlorophyll into hemoglobin, although it is not known exactly how this is done. Some scientists believe that humans may have the same ability.

We do know that chlorophyll builds up the amount of red blood cells in the bloodstream; it also strengthens the cells, detoxifies the liver and bloodstream, and chemically neutralizes polluting elements that can cause cancer.

Leafy green vegetables are the best source of chlorophyll. These include lettuce, kale, collards, Swiss chard, alfalfa, cabbage, spinach, watercress, parsley, celery, cucumbers, scallions, green peppers, and buckwheat, sunflower, and turnip greens. All of these foods adapt well to blending.

As you can see, our mothers and grandmothers had the right idea when they said, "Eat your vegetables," because these items are full of many of the nutrients our bodies need, and few of the less useful elements. If you go a step further and *blend* your vegetables, you will be sure of getting the maximum benefit from them. Once you become familiar with the desirable properties each food contains, it will be easy to assemble a nourishing and tasty assortment of vegetables, fruits, and grains for blending.

4

The Basics of Blending

There are a few terms and procedures in this book that may not be familiar to you if you are embarking on a living foods lifestyle for the first time. This chapter offers some helpful hints and suggestions to make blending and living foods even easier and more enjoyable. I will also explain some of the ways I have developed to get the maximum nutritional value from natural foods, and how these ways are applied in the recipes in this book. As I explain elsewhere, the recipe section is something in the nature of a "starter kit." When you have had more experience in blending, you will find satisfaction in working out your own combinations to produce delicious and satisfying meals that please your palate and meet your nutritional needs perfectly. If you are already familiar with the living foods lifestyle, you should read this chapter anyway; you may find some valuable suggestions that will enhance your blending experience even further.

SOME OF THE FOODS YOU WILL USE

"Living foods" are those that are uncooked, so their nutrient value is unchanged. When we eat living foods, we get the maximum amount of vitamins, minerals, enzymes, and other important nutrients in these foods, just as nature intended. Living foods include sprouts, greens, fresh fruits and vegetables, sea vegetables, and naturally fermented foods.

When we talk about "leafy green vegetables," we are referring to lettuce, escarole, endive, spinach, Swiss chard, watercress, and dandelion, mustard, turnip, and beet greens. As you have seen in the previous chapter, these are all excellent sources of chlorophyll, as well as calcium, iron, and many vitamins. "Root vegetables" include carrots, parsnips, rutabagas, onions, and beets. "Indoor greens," including sunflower greens and buckwheat lettuce, are used in many of the recipes in this book. For those who are not familiar with them, they are seven-day-old greens, four to five inches tall, that are grown indoors from whole seeds on an inch of soil.

Many of the recipes in this book call for soaked dried fruits. Unless the soaking time is specified in the recipe, dried fruits should be soaked in just enough spring or filtered water to cover them until they are soft. The amount of time required depends on the fruit; raisins, for example, take about one hour. In some cases, fruits must be soaked overnight. The water in which fruits were soaked can be reserved and used to flavor your recipes.

The soy products—tofu, miso, tempeh, and tamari —have become very popular in recent years. They are all very healthy, as well as useful. Tofu is a mild bean curd made from soaked soybeans, with the liquid drained off and the solids allowed to set. Miso is fermented soybean paste. The three most popular varieties are natto, mugi, and kome, or rice miso. Tempeh is made from partially cooked, fermented soybeans, and is the richest known source of vitamin B_{12}. Tamari is a naturally fermented sauce made from soybeans. It is more concentrated than regular soy sauce, which usually contains sugar or preservatives and MSG.

Seaweed has also become a popular addition to many modern diets. Nori, which is obtainable from health food stores in thin sheets, is high in protein, vitamin B_{12}, and vitamin C. Dulse, a purplish-red variety, is high in iron, potassium, and sodium. Wakame, a member of the kelp family, is high in calcium. Kanten, also known as agar-agar, is a translucent, chunky variety. It contains no protein, fat, or carbohydrates, but it does have some calcium and a little iodine. It is a replacement for gelatin in some desserts, and is also a natural laxative. Hiziki, which comes in dark strands, and arame are both useful and palatable additions to salads. Kelp, which is used in many of the recipes in this book, is available raw, but it is usually sold dried and granulated or ground into powder. It can be used as a condiment or salt substitute. It is an excellent source of vitamins—especially the B complex—and essential minerals and enzymes.

In addition to being high in many nutrients, seaweed contains alginic acid, which gives it the ability to help discharge heavy metals, including radioactive wastes, from the body in the form of insoluble salts.

Legumes are a valuable addition to the diet. Most people are familiar with kidney, pinto, and navy beans, but you should not overlook black beans, chickpeas (also known as garbanzo beans), and adzuki beans. These are the least fatty of all beans, and the most readily digestible.

Seeds to be blended should include the readily available sesame and sunflower seeds, as well as pine nuts (also called pignoli). If seeds or nuts are to be soaked before using, put them in just enough spring or filtered water to cover them. They are usually left overnight unless otherwise specified in the recipe. Unlike the soaking water from dried fruits, this water should not be reused in recipes because of its chemical content. Both seeds and legumes may also be used in their sprouted form; sprouting neutralizes the natural enzyme inhibitors in beans, seeds, nuts, and grains, so even more enzymes are available for your body's use.

Seed and nut meals are easily made at home by grinding the seeds or nuts, ¼ cup at a time, in a small hand grinder or in a blender at high speed. These meals are useful as thickeners and are often used as a substitute for wheat flour.

Free Food for the Harvesting

All around us are plants that, if we exercise a little caution in our choices, can provide us with food that is free except for the labor of obtaining it. These "field plants" are rich in vitamins, minerals, and other nutrients the body needs for good health. They are largely regarded as weeds in this country, but in many rural areas overseas, they have long been part of the diet. These include:

- Dandelions: *If they are picked while young, before the flowers have formed, dandelions are rich in vitamins A and D, and in minerals such as calcium, manganese, chlorine, potassium, and iron. Earlier generations were very familiar with dandelion tea, made from an infusion of the young plants.*

- Purslane: *This is a very tasty succulent, rich in iron, calcium, and vitamin A.*

- Lamb's quarters: *Like dandelions, this plant should be picked while it is young, before the flowers have formed. It is rich in vitamins A and C, and also has a high content of thiamin, riboflavin, and niacin.*

- Chickweed: *This plant grows in cultivated fields. It helps to increase the absorptive ability of all membranes, and to eliminate congestion; it is also good for the liver, kidneys, and lungs. Chickweed contains B complex vitamins, vitamin C, beta-carotene, magnesium, iron, calcium, and many other nutrients.*

- Watercress: *This can be found in many streams. It is excellent for convalescence. Watercress is a good source of B complex vitamins, vitamins A, C, and E, as well as iron, calcium, phosphorus, and other minerals.*

- Chicory: *The blue flowers of this plant can be seen in waste land everywhere, and the young leaves can be added to your larder. The ancient Romans added chicory to their diet for kidney, liver, or stomach disorders.*

- Milkweed: *This looks similar to asparagus, and has white and purple-shaded flowers. Every part of this plant is edible. It is a good source of vitamin C and beta-carotene.*

- Amaranth: *This has been used as a food for centuries. It grows wild in the United States, but has only recently made an appearance in health food stores. It is full of vitamins, especially C, E, and some of the B complex. It is also an excellent source of protein.*

- Kudzu: *This is another roadside "weed," which has spread rapidly enough to be a nuisance of immense proportions in some parts of the country. However, it is a useful natural thickener, and we at the Foundation use it as such, similar to our use of avocado.*

Remember to always use common sense when picking field plants. Do not pick plants that grow by the roadside; these can be contaminated with pollution from passing cars, as well as by people who walk their dogs by the side of the road. Make sure the area where you pick the plants has not been treated with any kind of pesticides, as these can cause numerous health problems.

WHY BUY ORGANIC?

I recommend organically grown produce for blending for several reasons. One is that organic foods are "Earth-friendly;" that is, the soil, water, and air are not polluted because organic farmers do not use chemical fertilizers and pesticides. Because of this, organic foods are also "people-friendly." Foods treated with pesticides and other chemicals can cause many illnesses, including an increased risk of cancer. Also, some produce is irradiated in order to make it last longer in the store; this can cause health problems, as well.

If possible, try to buy produce that is grown in your area. Locally grown fruits and vegetables are usually picked at the peak of ripeness, and contain maximum nutritional value. Produce that is shipped in from another area is usually picked before it is completely ripe; this makes it last a little longer, but reduces the nutritional value.

BLENDING EQUIPMENT

You may use any type of blender for the recipes in this book, provided it has a strong motor and stainless steel blades. Some people prefer plastic pitchers because they are lightweight, but others feel there is a chance for contamination from plastic, and will only use glass pitchers. In any case, look for a blender with a wide-mouth pitcher, which is easiest to clean. A pitcher with markings for easy measurement is also helpful. A good, medium-priced blender with a strong motor usually costs about $35 to $45. Try to avoid the cheaper models with weaker motors; they tend to burn out quickly, and end up costing you more money. At the Ann Wigmore Foundation, we use a Vita-Mix blender; I have found that this is the best blender to use in the long run.

A Champion juicer is useful for making *Vegekraut* and several other recipes. However, a regular food processor will work just as well.

Sprout bags are used to make seed cheese. They are white, 8" by 12" drawstring bags made of special non-resinated nylon mesh. They are lightweight, highly durable, and machine washable. Sprout bags can be obtained from the Ann Wigmore Foundation by calling (617) 267-9424.

BLENDING CAUTIONS

Blending is a simple way to obtain the nutrition you need in an easy-to-digest form. In addition to following the recipes in this book, you should feel free to experiment with blending different foods to satisfy your personal tastes as well as your nutritional needs. In general, any type of living food adapts well to blending. However, there are a few things you should be aware of before you begin.

Some parts of certain foods should not be blended. The skins of oranges and grapefruits contain toxic substances, as do carrot and rhubarb greens. Always remove the pits and cores of fruits, especially apples, peaches, and plums; the seeds and pits of these fruits contain cyanide.

Whether it is organically grown or not, all produce should be washed before using. Leave the peel on if the produce is organically grown, since most nutrients are located right under the skin, and are lost if the peel is removed. Some fruits and vegetables (such as apples and cucumbers) that are not organic are waxed to preserve their color, and the wax is not removed by washing. In this case, the produce should be peeled. Papayas should always be peeled, since they are often grown in tropical countries using pesticides that are banned in the United States.

Always cut fruits and vegetables into slices or chunks before blending them. This will make it easier on your blender's motor and blades.

REJUVELAC AND OTHER BASICS

Most of the recipes in this book include *Rejuvelac* as an ingredient, to be blended with vegetables or fruits to obtain a smooth texture. *Rejuvelac* is a slightly fermented wheatberry drink that is one of the most important items in the living foods lifestyle. *Rejuvelac* contains a very high level of enzymes that help you properly digest food, and replaces the enzymes that are lost in cooked foods. Because one of the biggest health problems is a deficiency of enzymes, *Rejuvelac* plays a vital role in restoring health. But that is only the beginning. As you know, wheat is one of the most nutritious foods known to man. *Rejuvelac* contains all the nutritional nourishment of wheat and is more easily digested. It contains the friendly bacteria that are necessary for a healthy colon and to remove toxins. It is also filled with B complex vitamins and vitamins C and E. Vitamin E is sometimes called a "youth vitamin;" it is believed to prevent premature aging by prolonging the life of our cells. It also helps prevent some aging-related degenerative diseases.

Rejuvelac prevents the oxidation of food when it is blended. Oxidation is a chemical reaction that breaks down food; this occurs within the body as a natural part of digestion, and in this case, the nutrition and energy contained in the food is utilized to our benefit. However, when oxidation occurs outside the body, the nutrients in food are damaged or destroyed, and are therefore of little or no benefit to us.

Harvey Lisle, a food chemist who has worked extensively with sprouted grains, has this to say about *Rejuvelac:* "For a seed to sprout, three key ingredients or forces are required: water or moisture, warmth, and sun forces. It may be argued that seeds in the soil do not get the visible sunshine, but there are sun forces that are not visible, as found in the infrared and ultraviolet spectrums. With these forces working on the seed, it breaks out of dormancy and starts to sprout. These forces enliven the seed's minerals and vitamins; the minerals become available and the vitamins increase by several hundred percent. The sprouts then impart these vital forces to the water used to make *Rejuvelac.* Swirling the sprouts in the *Rejuvelac* for several minutes before drinking it helps to transfer the sprouts' vital forces to the water. Then, as you drink the *Rejuvelac,* you are taking these vital forces into your own system.

"To understand what is taking place in the *Rejuvelac,* think of grapes. Grapes can be made into grape juice or wine, which is fermented grape juice. We take the sprouted wheat and make it into sprouted wheat juice, which is basically what you drink after the second or third day. Fermentation, which can be detected by flavor changes, starts at about that time, depending upon the temperature; by the fourth and fifth day the *Rejuvelac,* along with its sprouts, should be discarded, since the sprouts are now rapidly losing their life and forces.

"I have observed the use of sprouts in other dietary applications. Sprouts, through their new emerging growth, manifest the forces of youth and growth. By eating the sprouts or drinking the *Rejuvelac,* we, too, can benefit from these forces."

Fermentation is an important factor in aiding digestion through nourishing enzymes. During fermentation, complex proteins, starches, and fats in food are broken into simple compounds called predigested foods, that are easily assimilated by the body with a minimum of effort and energy. In the living foods lifestyle, *Rejuvelac* is the most widely used of the fermented foods. Others include *Vegekraut* and fermented seed dishes, creams, and milks, all of which are described in this section, and are used in many of the recipes in the recipe section. They are rich in enzymes, predigested protein, and lactic acid, and aid the ready digestion of food even when there has been a minimum of chewing.

MAKING REJUVELAC

Preparation of *Rejuvelac* is simple, but it does take some time, so it must be made in advance. You will need a clean, wide-mouth glass jar, measuring one-half or one gallon; a piece of nylon mesh or cheesecloth; a supply of soft wheatberries (spring wheat); and a strong rubber band.

Fill the jar one-fourth full of wheatberries. Cover the mouth of the jar with nylon mesh or cheesecloth, and secure the mesh with a strong rubber band. Add enough spring or filtered water to fill the jar. Allow the wheatberries to soak for eight to ten hours, then drain them, rinse, and drain again. Place the jar at an angle so that the berries continuously drain. Make sure that the wheatberries do not completely cover the mouth of the jar, because they will need ventilation. The wheatberries will start to sprout. Rinse them about two or three times a day during the sprouting stage. After two days, rinse the sprouted wheatberries thoroughly for the last time. Drain off the rinsing water, fill the jar to the top with spring or filtered water, and allow the sprouts to soak for forty-eight hours. At the end of this time, this soaking liquid is your first batch of *Rejuvelac*. Pour this off into another jar for immediate use or keep it in the refrigerator to slow down the fermentation process.

Refill the jar with the same amount of spring or filtered water to make your second batch of *Rejuvelac*, but this time soak the sprouts for only twenty-four hours. Pour off this second batch and refill the jar with the same amount of spring or filtered water to make the final batch of *Rejuvelac*. Again, soak the sprouts for only twenty-four hours. After you have made three batches, feed the spent wheatberries to the birds.

Good *Rejuvelac* is a cloudy, slightly yellow liquid, with a tart, lemonade flavor. When it is fermented too long, it can become very sour. Since it is constantly fermenting, it is natural that tiny bubbles rise through the liquid occasionally. The very best *Rejuvelac* is in fact slightly carbonated. It is also natural for a layer of white foam to form on top of the *Rejuvelac*. This is not harmful and can be used. *Rejuvelac* can be kept in the refrigerator for a few days to a week, as long as the taste is still agreeable to you. Drink *Rejuvelac* before or between meals to avoid diluting the digestive juices after a meal.

SUNFLOWER SEED CHEESE

Seed cheese is a very concentrated food, and should be used in moderation; I don't take more than four table-spoons at a time myself. Seed cheese provides valuable fats, predigested protein, B complex vitamins, vitamin E, calcium, iron, phosphorus, potassium, and magnesium.

To make seed cheese, soak hulled sunflower seeds in spring or filtered water for four to five hours. Drain and rinse. Fill the blender about half full with the seeds, and add enough *Rejuvelac* to cover the seeds by about an inch. Blend into a smooth, creamy texture. If neces-sary, add more *Rejuvelac*. Pour the mixture into a sprout bag (see page 35) or a piece of cheesecloth and hang the bag over a bowl to drain for about three to four hours. The outer layer will turn slightly dark because it has been exposed to the air. If it becomes extremely dark, skim off this layer. Place the contents in a glass jar or a container with a lid, and pack down to remove any air pockets. Cover the jar. Seed cheese will keep in the refrigerator for two to three days.

For variety, you can also use sesame or pumpkin seeds. Soak sesame seeds for five to six hours, and pumpkin seeds for eight hours. Try a mixture of dif-ferent seeds, such as 1 cup of sunflower seeds with 4 tablespoons of sesame seeds. Or even blend ½ cup chopped vegetables, like broccoli or cauliflower, with 1 cup of seeds.

ALMOND CREAM

Soak 1 cup of almonds in spring or filtered water for twenty-four hours, changing the soaking water twice. The almonds will almost double in size. After twenty-four hours, discard the water. In order to remove the skins, heat some water until it is nearly boiling and put the almonds in for only five to ten seconds. Remove the almonds from the heat, pour into a strainer, and immediately run cold water on them to prevent them from cooking. Pop the almonds out of their skins, and discard the skins.

Put the almonds into the blender and fill with *Rejuvelac* or spring or filtered water to two inches above the almonds. Blend to a very creamy consistency. If necessary, add more liquid. Be sure to blend the mixture well, or the small particles could get caught in your throat. Put the cream in a container with a lid and store in the refrigerator. This will make about 1½ cups. Stronger *Rejuvelac* makes a stronger almond cream, and weaker *Rejuvelac* makes a mild almond cream. If you use spring or filtered water instead of *Rejuvelac*, let the almond cream sit at room temperature for three to four hours so that it can ferment. After fermentation, keep the almond cream in the refrigerator; it will keep for three to four days.

ALMOND MILK

Almond milk is an excellent substitute for cow's milk. It is a refreshing and substantial between-meals drink that is usually very popular with children.

To make almond milk, take 3 to 4 tablespoons of almond cream, made as described above, mix it with approximately 1 cup *Rejuvelac*, and blend for about five seconds. This will make a light milk, but you may add more or less *Rejuvelac*, depending on the flavor you want. A richer milk can be made by blending 1 cup of almond cream with 1 cup of *Rejuvelac*. Place the mixture in a sprout bag, and squeeze out the liquid. This liquid will be similar in consistency to cow's milk.

The taste of almond milk improves after a day or so. It will keep for three to four days in the refrigerator.

VEGEKRAUT

Vegekraut is a fermented mixture of several root vegetables that are ordinarily hard to digest, such as carrots, beets, cauliflower, cabbage, and potatoes. Fermentation, however, releases the enzymes and makes these vegetables more digestible. *Vegekraut* should consist of about 80 percent cabbage to 20 percent other vegetables.

Reserve three or four outer leaves from the cabbage. You will need a food processor to grate or shred the cabbage and other vegetables. A Champion juicer (with blank attachment for food processing) is perfect for this. Process the vegetables until the juice flows; the more juice, the better. Place the mixture in a crock or a wide-mouth glass jar, leaving a little room for expansion. Cover the mixture with the reserved cabbage leaves and place a plate on top of the leaves. Place something heavy on the plate to weigh the contents down. Cover the entire crock or jar with a towel or cloth, and let this sit at room temperature for about three to five days. A warmer climate will mean faster fermentation. A cooler climate means slower fermentation.

When the *Vegekraut* is fermented, remove the weight, the plate, and the cabbage leaves. If you like the cabbage leaves, you may eat them. Usually, the top layer of the *Vegekraut* will be slightly darker than the rest. If the taste of this layer is not disagreeable to you, it is fine to eat. There will be juice near the surface of the *Vegekraut*. Take a long wooden spoon and mix the juice in well. Transfer the *Vegekraut* to a clean glass jar, cover, and store in the refrigerator. It will keep anywhere from a few weeks to a month. It can be eaten alone, added to *Rejuvelac* to make a tangy drink, or added to soups.

5

Blended Drinks

A variety of thirst-quenching, cooling, and nutritious drinks will be at your fingertips once you become accustomed to using your blender and juicer to maximum capacity. You will learn to combine various ingredients to produce a wide range of drinks that will satisfy your taste buds as well as provide essential nutrients. These energy drinks are easy to digest and have proved helpful in overcoming the craving for sweets that many starting on the living foods lifestyle experience. Make the drinks that appeal to you two or three times daily for about three weeks, and you'll find you no longer crave the sweets or junk foods that you once thought were essential. You can always add a couple of soaked dates or a little raw honey if it is necessary to sweeten the drink slightly.

While these drinks are suitable for everyone, they especially appeal to children. Children who are being started on the right road to health with the living foods lifestyle often look for something light, flavorful, and satisfying—try the "smoothies" in this chapter.

More or less *Rejuvelac* can be added, depending on whether you want a smoothie or a thinner drink. When the drink is made with *Rejuvelac*, it will last a day or two, since the *Rejuvelac* contains vitamin E, which acts as an antioxidant. The leftover drink should be kept in the refrigerator. If the drink is made with water, it must be used immediately.

APPLE-BANANA DRINK

Yield: 1 serving

1 apple, peeled, cored, and sliced
1 cup *Rejuvelac* (page 38) or spring water
2 bananas, sliced

1. Blend the apple with the *Rejuvelac* or spring water. Add the bananas, and blend again.

2. Pour into a tall glass and serve.

APPLE-KIWI DRINK

Yield: 1 serving

2 apples, peeled, cored, and sliced
2 kiwis, peeled
½ cup *Rejuvelac* (page 38) or spring water

1. Blend all the ingredients together until smooth.

2. Pour into a tall glass and serve.

BANANA SMOOTHIE

Yield: Approximately 1 cup

½ cup soaked dried apricots

1 cup *Rejuvelac* (page 38) or spring water
in which apricots were soaked

1 banana

1. Blend the apricots with the *Rejuvelac* or the water.

2. Add the banana and give the blender a final short
burst for a smooth-textured drink.

3. Pour into tall glasses and serve.

CAROB SMOOTHIE

Yield: Approximately 1 to 2 cups

½ cup pitted dates

½ cup coconut, in pieces or shredded

5 tablespoons carob powder

1 cup *Rejuvelac* (page 38) or spring water

1 banana (optional)

1. Blend the dates, coconut, carob powder, and *Rejuvelac*
or spring water together until smooth.

2. Blend in the banana if a thicker smoothie is wanted.

3. Pour into tall glasses and serve.

CARROT-AVOCADO DRINK

Yield: 1 serving

2 cups carrot juice
1 medium avocado, peeled and chopped

1. Blend all the ingredients together until smooth.
2. Pour into a tall glass and serve.

CITRUS DRINK

Yield: Approximately 2 cups

2 oranges, peeled and seeded
1 tablespoon honey
1 cup *Rejuvelac* (page 38) or spring water
1 small avocado, peeled and sliced, if necessary

1. Blend the oranges with the honey and *Rejuvelac* or spring water.
2. If you want a thicker "smoothie," blend in the avocado.
3. Pour into tall glasses and serve.

COCONUT DRINK

Yield: Approximately 1½ cups

1 cup shredded coconut

½ cup coconut milk or apple juice

¼ teaspoon ground ginger, or
1 teaspoon chopped fresh ginger

1 tablespoon honey

1. Blend all the ingredients together until smooth.

2. Pour into tall glasses and serve.

GREEN DRINK

Yield: Approximately 4 cups

A Champion juicer must be used for this recipe, rather than a blender, since there is no liquid added. Spice up this drink with your choice of flavorings, such as ginger or cinnamon—some people even like a dash of cayenne pepper.

1 cup buckwheat lettuce

1 cup sunflower greens

1 cup alfalfa sprouts

1 carrot, diced

1 stalk celery, diced

Your choice of spices to taste

1. Run all the ingredients through the juicer.

2. Pour into tall glasses and serve.

MANGO DRINK

Yield: Approximately 2½ cups

2 ripe mangoes, sliced
½ cup *Rejuvelac* (page 38) or spring water
3 ripe persimmons, sliced

1. Blend all the ingredients together until smooth.

2. Pour into tall glasses and serve.

PAPAYA-BANANA DRINK

Yield: 4 cups

2 cups peeled, seeded, and chopped papaya
2 cups sliced bananas
1–2 cups *Rejuvelac* (page 38) or spring water

1. Put the papaya and bananas in the blender. Add just
   enough *Rejuvelac* or spring water to cover the fruit,
   and blend until smooth.

2. Pour into tall glasses and serve.

PEACH SMOOTHIE

Yield: Approximately 2 cups

4 peaches, stones and skin removed
½ teaspoon ground ginger
½ cup shredded coconut
1 cup *Rejuvelac* (page 38) or spring water

1. Blend all the ingredients together until smooth.
2. Pour into tall glasses and serve.

PINEAPPLE-BANANA DRINK

Yield: 1 serving

2 cups diced pineapple
1 banana, sliced
½ cup *Rejuvelac* (page 38) or spring water

1. Blend all the ingredients together until smooth.
2. Pour into a tall glass and serve.

VEGEKRAUT BEVERAGE

Yield: Approximately 4 cups

This is a nutritious summertime thirst quencher, great for taking along on picnics.

1 cup *Rejuvelac* (page 38) or spring water
3–4 tablespoons *Vegekraut* (page 42)
Additional quart of
Rejuvelac (page 38) or spring water

1. Blend the cup of *Rejuvelac* or spring water and the *Vegekraut*.

2. Strain the mixture into the additional quart of *Rejuvelac* or spring water; pour into tall glasses and serve, or keep in the refrigerator for up to a day or two.

WATERMELON REFRESHER

Yield: Approximately 3 cups

This is a great "wake-up" morning drink.

4 cups watermelon strips,
with rind left on if organically grown

1. Put the watermelon strips through the Champion juicer.

2. Pour into tall glasses and serve.

WATERMELON SMOOTHIE

Yield: Approximately 2 cups

2 cups chopped watermelon, rind
and seeds removed

½ cup *Rejuvelac* (page 38) or spring water

1 small avocado, peeled and chopped

1. Gradually blend the watermelon with the *Rejuvelac* or spring water.

2. Blend in the avocado.

3. Pour into tall glasses and serve.

WATERMELON-AVOCADO DRINK

Yield: 1 serving

2 cups chopped watermelon,
with rind left on if organically grown

1 medium avocado, peeled and sliced

1. Put the watermelon in the blender, and blend until the juice flows.

2. Add the avocado, and blend until smooth.

3. Pour into a tall glass and serve.

6

Soups and Chowders

Soups provide the perfect nourishment for anyone who has trouble chewing or difficulty digesting large meals. Since the first step to digestion takes place in the mouth when saliva starts breaking down the starches in food, it is important to remember that, even though these soups have been blended till they are liquid or near-liquid in form, they should still be "chewed" in order to begin the breaking-down process that aids digestion.

Soups can be complete meals in themselves, or they can be used to "bulk up" a small meal when they are served as the first course. They are also economical, since small amounts of available ingredients can be used to produce a substantial serving. Variety is easily achieved by using different combinations of vegetables and different seasonings. High-energy nourishment can be provided by blending an assortment of sprouts, greens, and vegetables, and you can experiment further by including fruits such as chopped apples or watermelon.

Organically grown sprouts of various seeds are the ideal basic ingredients for energy soups, since they are high in enzymes and the other nutrients we need. Fortunately, stores that stock organically grown produce are opening in increasing numbers throughout the country in response to growing demand, so in most areas it is usually easy to get such things as kelp, dulse, avocados, watercress, parsley, and sprouts, as well as more traditional soup vegetables. And don't forget to acquaint yourself with the "free foods" mentioned on page 32, that are available in rural and semi-rural areas, just for the taking. Many of them can add that little touch of flavor to a blended soup that will provide the variety most of us need in our diet. Different combinations of vegetables and different seasonings will result in a varied, healthy intake that will give you the energy you need for your all daily activities.

ASPARAGUS SOUP
—VARIATION #1

Yield: Approximately 3 cups

1 cup chopped asparagus

1 cup *Rejuvelac* (page 38) or spring water

1 stalk celery, chopped

2 tablespoons chopped parsley

1 teaspoon kelp

1 small avocado, peeled and sliced

1. Blend all the ingredients, except the avocado, together.

2. Add the avocado, and blend until smooth.

3. Pour into soup bowls and serve.

ASPARAGUS SOUP
—VARIATION #2

Yield: Approximately 5 cups

1 cup chopped asparagus
(reserve a few tips for garnish)

1 cup *Rejuvelac* (page 38) or spring water

1 stalk celery, chopped

2 cups sunflower greens or buckwheat lettuce

2 sprigs parsley, minced

½ cup almond meal

1. Blend all the ingredients, adding the almond meal gradually at the last. Use more *Rejuvelac* or spring water if a thinner consistency is wanted.

2. Pour into soup bowls, garnish with the reserved asparagus, and serve.

ALMOND SOUP

Yield: Approximately 2 cups

1 cup almonds, soaked for 24 hours,
outer skins removed (see page 40)

1 cup *Rejuvelac* (page 38) or spring water

1 tablespoon sunflower seed meal

1 teaspoon freshly ground ginger

1. Blend all the ingredients together for 2 minutes.

2. Either pour into soup bowls and serve immediately or put into a jar, cover, and allow the mixture to ferment overnight.

AVOCADO CHOWDER

Yield: Approximately 3 cups

1 small onion, chopped
½ cup grated carrot
½ cup grated celery
1 small bell pepper, chopped
½ cup grated cabbage
1 tablespoon kelp
½ cup *Rejuvelac* (page 38) or spring water
1 avocado, peeled and diced

1. Blend all the ingredients, except the avocado, together in very short bursts, to produce a thick, chowdery texture.

2. Mix the diced avocado into the chowder mixture, pour into soup bowls, and serve.

AVOCADO SOUP

Yield: Approximately 3 cups

1 cup *Rejuvelac* (page 38) or spring water
1 cup any kind of sprouts
2 cups any kind of green vegetables, chopped
1 medium avocado, sliced

1. Blend all the ingredients, except the avocado, together until smooth.

2. Add the avocado, and blend until smooth.

3. Pour into soup bowls and serve.

BASIC SEED SOUP

Yield: Approximately 2½ cups

The basic seed soup recipe given below will serve as a "starter" for anyone who is new to the living foods lifestyle. As you become experienced and more confident, you will find that an enormous variety of changes can be made to avoid any possibility of monotony creeping into the diet.

½ cup sprouted seeds
(such as sunflower or pumpkin)

1 cup *Rejuvelac* (page 38) or spring water

1 cup sunflower greens, buckwheat lettuce,
or any kind of green vegetable

1 summer squash or zucchini, peeled
(if not organic), seeded, and grated

1. Presoak the seeds in spring water for approximately 8 hours. Drain, then blend with the *Rejuvelac* or spring water.

2. Add the greens and blend again.

3. Put the grated squash into a bowl, pour the blended mixture over it, and serve.

Variations

If a thicker-textured soup is wanted, blend in a small, cut-up avocado, or add the avocado to the bowl with the squash.

Use different types of greens or sprouts—try ¼ cup radish sprouts for a tangy taste, or ½ cup fenugreek sprouts, or substitute indoor greens for the sprouts.

BEET SOUP

Yield: Approximately 2 cups

1 large beet, sliced

1 cup *Rejuvelac* (page 38) or spring water

Juice of 1 lemon

½ avocado, peeled and sliced

2 teaspoons *Vegekraut* (page 42)

Chopped sunflower greens

1. Blend the beet with the *Rejuvelac* or spring water until creamy.

2. Add the lemon juice and the avocado.

3. Just before serving, add the *Vegekraut*. Serve over the chopped sunflower greens.

BROCCOLI SOUP

Yield: Approximately 2½ cups

1 cup chopped broccoli

1 cup *Rejuvelac* (page 38) or spring water

½ teaspoon kelp

1 cup alfalfa sprouts

1 avocado, peeled and sliced

Sliced mushrooms or chopped parsley
for garnish (optional)

1. Blend all the ingredients, except the avocado, together until smooth.

2. Add the avocado, and blend until smooth.

3. Pour into soup bowls, garnish with sliced mushrooms or chopped parsley, if desired, and serve.

BUCKWHEAT SPINACH SOUP

Yield: Approximately 2½ cups

2 cups chopped buckwheat lettuce

1 cup chopped sweet apple

1 cup *Rejuvelac* (page 38) or spring water

1 cup chopped spinach

2 teaspoons kelp

1 medium tomato, chopped

1 small avocado, chopped

1 tablespoon grated carrot for garnish

1. Reserve 1 cup chopped buckwheat lettuce.

2. Blend the remaining ingredients, except the avocado, together until creamy.

3. Add the avocado, and blend again.

4. Pour the soup into bowls, sprinkle with the reserved buckwheat lettuce and the grated carrot, and serve.

CACTUS SOUP

Yield: Approximately 3 cups

The older the cactus plant, the thicker the hardened outer skin, and it is necessary to peel down to the soft areas beneath if no young plants are available. If young, fresh cacti are at hand, they need hardly any peeling at all. If watermelon rind is not available, you can use broccoli stems with the hard outer skin peeled away, instead.

1 cup *Rejuvelac* (page 38) or spring water
½ cup peeled and cut-up soft cactus flesh
1 cup chopped watermelon rind, if available
1 cup greens, such as buckwheat
sprouts, okra, or others
1 tablespoon whole dulse, or
1 teaspoon powdered dulse
1 small avocado, peeled and chopped

1. Put the *Rejuvelac* or spring water into the blender, add the cactus and the rind, and then the greens and the dulse. Blend for a moment.

2. Add the avocado and blend until smooth, adding more liquid if necessary.

3. Pour into soup bowls and serve.

CARROT SOUP
—VARIATION #1

Yield: Approximately 3 cups

2 cups grated carrots

1 stalk celery, chopped

1½ cups *Rejuvelac* (page 38) or spring water

¼ teaspoon tamari or kelp

2 small avocados, peeled and sliced

1. Blend the carrots and celery with the *Rejuvelac* or spring water.

2. Add the tamari or kelp, then the avocado, and blend well.

3. Pour into soup bowls and serve.

CARROT SOUP
—VARIATION #2

Yield: Approximately 3½ cups

1 cup sliced carrots

1 cup *Rejuvelac* (page 38) or spring water

1 cup chopped celery

1 teaspoon tamari

1 cup chopped cabbage

1 red bell pepper, chopped

1 medium avocado, sliced

1. Blend all the ingredients, except the avocado, together.

2. Add the avocado, and blend until smooth.

3. Pour into soup bowls and serve.

CARROT AND PEA SOUP

Yield: Approximately 3–4 cups

2 cups sliced carrots

2 cups *Rejuvelac* (page 38) or spring water

1 cup sprouted green peas

1/3 clove garlic

2 stalks celery, diced

1/2 teaspoon kelp

Alfalfa sprouts for garnish

1. Blend all the ingredients together, except the sprouts.

2. Pour into soup bowls, garnish with the alfalfa sprouts, and serve.

CASHEW SOUP

Yield: Approximately 2 cups

1/2 cup soaked cashews

1 cup *Rejuvelac* (page 38) or spring water

1 teaspoon kelp or dulse

Juice of 1 lemon

1/2 teaspoon paprika

2 cups chopped watercress

1. Blend all the ingredients together until smooth.

2. Pour into soup bowls and serve.

CAULIFLOWER SOUP

Yield: Approximately 2 cups

1 cup chopped cauliflower

1 cup *Rejuvelac* (page 38) or spring water

1 small zucchini, sliced

¼ cup minced parsley

1 avocado, sliced (optional)

1. Blend all the ingredients, except the avocado, together until smooth. Add the avocado if a thicker texture is desired.

2. Pour into soup bowls and serve.

CHICKPEA SOUP

Yield: Approximately 3 cups

1 cup chickpea sprouts

1½ cups *Rejuvelac* (page 38) or spring water

2 cups chopped sweet apple

3 tablespoons white dulse

Pine nuts for garnish (optional)

1. Blend the chickpea sprouts with the *Rejuvelac* or spring water, and add the apple and the dulse.

2. Serve over additional sprouts or pour into soup bowls, garnish with the pine nuts, and serve.

CELERY SOUP

2 small potatoes, diced

1 cup *Rejuvelac* (page 38) or spring water

2 stalks celery, diced
(reserve a few leaves for garnish)

$^1/_3$ cup diced onion

2 teaspoons chopped parsley

1 small zucchini, diced

1 cup grated carrot

1. Soak the potatoes in the *Rejuvelac* or spring water for 2 to 3 hours to soften the starch.

2. Blend the potatoes and the *Rejuvelac* or spring water with the celery for 10 seconds.

3. Add the onion, parsley, zucchini, and carrot, and blend until the desired consistency is reached.

4. Pour into soup bowls, garnish with the reserved celery leaves, and serve.

CORN CHOWDER

Yield: Approximately 5 cups

2 tomatoes, chopped

1 cup shredded zucchini

Kernels from 2 ears of corn

½ cup *Rejuvelac* (page 38) or spring water

½ cup celery juice

2 tablespoons chopped scallions

1 cup chopped carrots

½ green bell pepper, chopped

1 avocado, peeled and sliced

1. Reserve ¼ cup each of the tomatoes and zucchini.

2. Place the remaining tomatoes in the blender, and liquefy by turning the blender on and off several times.

3. Add the corn, *Rejuvelac* or spring water, celery juice, scallions, carrots, and pepper, and blend until smooth. Add the avocado, and blend again.

4. Pour the mixture into soup bowls, garnish with the reserved vegetables, and serve.

CORN SOUP

Vegetable seasoning is a mix of dehydrated vegetables and sea vegetables. It contains no salt or sugar, and is an excellent flavoring.

1 large ear fresh corn

1 cup *Rejuvelac* (page 38) or spring water

1 large tomato, sliced

1 teaspoon vegetable seasoning
(such as Bernard Jensen's vegetable seasoning)

2 green peppers, chopped

1 teaspoon minced parsley

1 teaspoon kelp

1 cup any kind of sprouts

1 avocado, peeled and chopped

1. Cut the corn from the cob, and reserve ¼ cup of the kernels.

2. Blend the remaining corn with the other ingredients, except the avocado, until smooth.

3. Add the avocado, and blend again.

4. Pour the mixture into soup bowls, garnish with the reserved corn, and serve.

CREAM OF BROCCOLI SOUP

Yield: Approximately 4 cups

3 cups broccoli, chopped

½ cup *Rejuvelac* (page 38) or spring water

1 cup chopped celery

½ cup chopped carrots

½ cup sprouted sunflower seeds,
or ½ cup soaked pine nuts

1. Blend all the ingredients, except the seeds or nuts, together until smooth.

2. Add the seeds or nuts, and blend again.

3. Pour into soup bowls and serve.

CREAM OF CARROT SOUP

Yield: Approximately 3 cups

2 cups chopped carrots

1 cup *Rejuvelac* (page 38) or spring water

1 stalk celery, chopped

2 large sprigs parsley, chopped

1 medium avocado, peeled and sliced

Grated carrot for garnish (optional)

1. Blend all the ingredients, except the avocado, together until smooth.

2. Add the avocado, and blend again.

3. Pour into soup bowls, garnish with grated carrot, if desired, and serve.

CREAM OF TOMATO SOUP —VARIATION #1

Yield: Approximately 3 cups

2 tomatoes, diced

1 sprig parsley, minced

½ cucumber, grated

1 stalk celery, chopped

2 red peppers, chopped

½ avocado, peeled and sliced

1. Place the tomatoes in the blender, and liquefy them by turning the blender on and off several times.

2. Add the remaining ingredients, except the avocado, and blend until smooth.

3. Add the avocado, and blend again.

4. Pour into soup bowls and serve.

CREAM OF TOMATO SOUP —VARIATION #2

Yield: Approximately 6 cups

Tomatillos are small, tomatolike fruits that can be brown, yellow, red, orange, or purple in color. If they are not available, you may use an extra tomato.

3 stalks celery, chopped

1 cup pine nuts (pignoli)

4 tomatoes, halved

4 tomatillos (if available)

6–8 sprigs fresh parsley

1. Reserve ¹/₃ of the chopped celery and a few nuts for garnish.

2. Place the tomatoes and tomatillos (if available) in the blender, and liquefy them by turning the blender on and off several times.

3. Add the parsley, celery, and nuts, and blend.

4. Pour into soup bowls, garnish with the reserved celery and nuts, and serve.

CREAMY AVOCADO SOUP

Yield: Approximately 2 cups

½ cup chopped celery

1 cup chopped parsley

1 cup mixed vegetables,
combining any of the following:
squash, carrots, spinach, cauliflower,
and beets

1 cup *Rejuvelac* (page 38) or spring water

1 avocado, peeled and sliced

1. Blend all the ingredients, except the avocado, together until smooth.

2. Add the avocado, and blend again.

3. Pour into soup bowls and serve.

CUCUMBER SOUP

Yield: Approximately 3 cups

1 apple, peeled, cored, and sliced
1 cucumber, peeled, seeded, and grated
1 small red pepper, seeded and chopped
2 cups almond or sunflower seed milk (page 41)
1 teaspoon kelp
½ cup soaked cashew nuts and
a few cucumber slices for garnish

1. Blend the apple, cucumber, and red pepper with the seed milk until well blended.

2. Pour into soup bowls, garnish with the cucumber slices, cashews, and kelp, and serve.

DULSE SOUP

Yield: Approximately 2 cups

¾ cup dulse
3 tomatoes, diced
¼ cup chopped chives
1 avocado, peeled and sliced

1. Blend all the ingredients, except the avocado, together until smooth.

2. Add the avocado, and blend until smooth.

3. Pour into soup bowls and serve.

ENERGY SOUP

Yield: Approximately 6 cups

This is a recipe that can be varied greatly, the combinations limited only by your imagination and tastes. For example, the amount and type of greens used can be varied. A great variety of different spices can be used to change the taste, such as nutmeg, cinnamon, and coriander. The amount of liquid (*Rejuvelac* or spring water) used depends on how thick or thin a texture you prefer, so this can be adjusted to your own taste. The *Rejuvelac* can add a tang if it has a little honey added, and is fermented at room temperature for two to three more days before using.

1 tablespoon dulse

2 cups *Rejuvelac* (page 38) or spring water

½ cup mixed sprouts

½ cup watermelon rind
(the white part, without the skin), optional

1 carrot, diced

2 cups edible wild greens, such as
lamb's quarters or purslane (see page 32)

4 cups chopped chlorophyll-rich greens, such as
sunflower greens, buckwheat lettuce,
or celery leaves

2 apples, peeled, cored, and quartered

1 avocado, peeled and sliced

1. Blend together the dulse, *Rejuvelac* or spring water, sprouts, watermelon rind if used, carrot, and wild greens.

2. Add the chlorophyll-rich greens and blend.

3. Add the apples and blend.

4. Add the avocado, and blend until smooth.

5. Pour the mixture into soup bowls and serve with cut-up bananas, alfalfa sprouts, or watermelon.

JERUSALEM ARTICHOKE SOUP

Yield: Approximately 3½ cups

1 cup sliced Jerusalem artichokes

1 cup *Rejuvelac* (page 38) or spring water

2 cups sliced carrots

1 avocado, peeled and sliced

1. Blend all the ingredients, except the avocado, together until smooth.

2. Add the avocado, and blend until smooth.

3. Pour into soup bowls and serve.

LENTIL SOUP

Yield: Approximately 3 cups

2 cups sprouted lentils

1 cup *Rejuvelac* (page 38) or spring water

½ cup buckwheat lettuce

½ cup any kind of seaweed

½ cup minced parsley

1 small avocado, peeled and sliced

1. Blend all the ingredients, except the avocado, together until smooth.

2. Add the avocado, and blend until smooth.

3. Pour into soup bowls and serve.

MUSHROOM SOUP

Yield: Approximately 3 cups

2 cups sliced mushrooms

1 cup *Rejuvelac* (page 38) or spring water

½ cup soaked cashews

½ cup sprouts (either alfalfa, red clover,
or radish, or a mixture of these)
or minced parsley

1. Blend all the ingredients together until smooth.

2. Pour into soup bowls and serve.

OKRA SOUP

Yield: Approximately 6 cups

2 cups chopped okra

½ cup *Rejuvelac* (page 38) or spring water

2 cups chopped carrots

1 tablespoon lemon juice

1 cup chopped zucchini

1 cup chopped celery

1 cup mung bean sprouts

¹/₈ teaspoon cayenne pepper

1. Blend all the ingredients together until smooth.

2. Pour into soup bowls and serve.

PEA SOUP

Yield: Approximately 3 cups

Any other dried fruit can be substituted for the prunes, but it should be presoaked before blending.

1 cup sprouted peas (dried peas should be
soaked and sprouted before use)

1 cup *Rejuvelac* (page 38) or spring water

2 cups okra

½ cup chopped, pitted prunes

2 large cabbage leaves, chopped

1. Blend all the ingredients together until smooth.

2. Pour into soup bowls and serve.

PUMPKIN SOUP

Yield: Approximately 4½ cups

2 cups chopped pumpkin

1 cup *Rejuvelac* (page 38) or spring water

1 tablespoon tamari

½ bell pepper, chopped

1 tablespoon kelp

1 tomato, chopped

1 stalk celery, chopped

½ avocado, peeled and sliced

1. Blend all the ingredients, except the avocado, together until smooth.

2. Add the avocado, and blend until smooth.

3. Pour into soup bowls and serve.

RADISH SPROUT SOUP

Yield: Approximately 2 cups

½ cup radish sprouts
½ cup *Rejuvelac* (page 38) or spring water
1 cup chopped celery
1 tablespoon kelp
Juice of ½ lemon
1 avocado, peeled, seeded, and sliced

1. Blend all the ingredients, except the avocado, together to the desired consistency.

2. Add the avocado, and blend again.

3. Serve over a bowl of radish sprouts.

RAINBOW SOUP

Yield: Approximately 4 cups

3 cups chopped tomatoes
½ cucumber, sliced
½ zucchini or yellow squash
¼ cup chopped celery
¼ cup chopped green pepper or cabbage
Dash each of basil, thyme, and cayenne pepper

1. Put the chopped tomatoes in the blender and turn the blender on and off several times to extract the juice from the tomatoes.

2. Add the remaining ingredients and blend until smooth.

3. Pour into soup bowls and serve.

SQUASH SOUP

Yield: Approximately 5 cups

4 medium tomatoes, chopped
2 cups grated zucchini
1 cup grated yellow squash
1 cup chopped dulse
1 cup *Rejuvelac* (page 38) or spring water
1 cup almond cream (page 40)

1. Reserve ½ cup of the mixed vegetables.

2. Blend the remaining vegetables with the dulse and *Rejuvelac* or spring water. Add the almond cream, and blend again.

3. Put the reserved vegetables into serving bowls, pour the blended mixture over them, and serve.

SWEET POTATO SOUP

Yield: Approximately 3 cups

1 sweet potato, sliced
1½ cups *Rejuvelac* (page 38) or spring water
1 cup carrot juice
Pinch each of nutmeg, kelp, and
cayenne pepper
1 avocado, peeled and sliced

1. Soak the sweet potato in the *Rejuvelac* or spring water for 2 to 3 hours, to soften the starch.

2. Blend the sweet potato and the *Rejuvelac* or spring water with the carrot juice and spices until smooth.

3. Add the avocado, and blend again.

4. Pour into soup bowls and serve.

SUMMER TREAT SOUP

Yield: Approximately 5 cups

2 large cucumbers, sliced

3 large tomatoes, diced

1 tablespoon chopped scallions

1 sweet red pepper, chopped

1 tablespoon kelp

1 tablespoon minced parsley or
watercress for garnish

1. Reserve a few cucumber slices for garnish.

2. Place the tomatoes in the blender, and liquefy them by turning the blender on and off several times.

3. Blend the remaining cucumber with the liquefied tomatoes, red pepper, kelp, and scallions until smooth.

4. Pour the mixture into soup bowls. Just before serving, add the reserved cucumber slices, but do not blend them in. Garnish with the parsley or the watercress, and serve.

STRING BEAN AND
TOMATO SOUP

Yield: Approximately 3 cups

10 string beans, sliced

1 cup *Rejuvelac* (page 38) or spring water

2 tomatoes, chopped

Juice of half a lemon

Dash cayenne pepper

½ cup celery juice

½ cup carrot juice

1 avocado, peeled and diced

1. Blend all the ingredients, except the avocado, together until smooth.

2. Add the avocado, and blend until smooth.

3. Pour into soup bowls and serve.

TOMATO SOUP

Yield: Approximately 2 cups

¼ cup sliced potato

½ cup *Rejuvelac* (page 38) or spring water

3 tomatoes, diced

½ cup carrot juice

¼ cup celery juice

½ teaspoon dried basil, or
3 tablespoons chopped fresh basil

1. Soak the sliced potato in the *Rejuvelac* or spring water for 2 to 3 hours to soften the starch.

2. Blend the potato and the *Rejuvelac* or spring water with the remaining ingredients until smooth. You may add more juice at the very end if the mixture is too hard to blend.

3. Pour into soup bowls and serve.

TOMATO AND CORN CHOWDER

Yield: Approximately 4 cups

¼ cup sunflower seeds

2 tomatoes, diced

½ cup *Rejuvelac* (page 38) or spring water

1 clove garlic

¼ cup chopped celery

Kernels from 3 ears corn

1. Soak the sunflower seeds for 5 to 6 hours, drain, and rinse.

2. Place the tomatoes in the blender, and liquefy them by turning the blender on and off several times.

3. Add the sunflower seeds and remaining ingredients. Blend until smooth and creamy.

4. Pour into soup bowls and serve.

ZUCCHINI SOUP
—VARIATION #1

Yield: Approximately 2 cups

1 small zucchini, grated
½ cup *Rejuvelac* (page 38) or spring water
1 stalk celery, chopped
4 sprigs parsley, chopped
1 cup any kind of sprouts
1 tablespoon tamari

1. Blend all the ingredients together until smooth.

2. Pour into soup bowls and serve.

ZUCCHINI SOUP
—VARIATION #2

Yield: Approximately 3 cups

2 cups diced zucchini
1 cup *Rejuvelac* (page 38) or spring water
1 cup buckwheat or sunflower greens
Kelp to taste
1 medium avocado, peeled and diced

1. Blend all the ingredients, except the avocado, together until smooth.

2. Add the avocado, and blend until smooth.

3. Pour into soup bowls and serve.

7

Sauces and Dressings

Nature has given us foods full of beautiful, natural seasonings, but because most of us have grown used to a diet rich in artificial seasonings, especially salts and sugars, we need to accustom ourselves and our palates to creative, natural sauce making. A wide range of sauces can be used to vary the living foods diet and step up the taste of the basic dishes, while still providing the essential nourishment that the body requires. We should attempt to make the transition from artificial seasonings to lighter sauces, containing sprouted seeds, nuts, and spices, in order to enjoy the true taste of natural foods.

This chapter contains recipes for basic sauces and dressings to get you started, but as any good cook will tell you, the most satisfying recipes are those you invent yourself, using your nose, your taste buds, and your imagination. As you add a little of this and a little of that, disregarding exact measurements and procedures, you allow your creative talents to come to the fore. You should regard each sauce as a new creation, and enjoy it when your friends try to guess what ingredients you have used.

HINTS FOR SAUCE MAKING

Here are a few basic suggestions, as well as hints on how to correct any problems you might encounter during your experiments with sauce making.

You will find *Rejuvelac* a great help when making sauces, but if you prefer to use spring or filtered water, that is fine, too. Some recipes may have specific fermenting times, but in general, if you use *Rejuvelac,* let your sauce ferment for six to eight hours; if you use water, the fermenting time should be fifteen to twenty hours. You will have to judge the time depending on how long the *Rejuvelac* was fermented when it was made, and the temperature of the room in which the sauce is being kept. Ideally, this should be from 68°F to 75°F, until fermentation takes place. Some recipes, such as Beet Sauce (page 89), contain neither water nor *Rejuvelac*. These should be fermented for just a few hours, according to your own taste. Fruit sauces should be fermented for about two to three hours, or until their flavor is rich, but not too strong.

If you use any oil in your recipes, I strongly recommend the use of pure, raw, cold-pressed olive oil. It is rich in chlorophyll, and thus ideal for food preparation. Other oils have usually been heat-treated, which makes them harder to digest and less healthy.

Sometimes, problems may arise when making sauces. For example, the end product may be too thick, too thin, or too sour for your individual taste. These problems are easily remedied. If the sauce is too thick, stir in a little more *Rejuvelac* or spring water. If it is too thin, grind up some seeds or nuts to make one or two tablespoons of meal, and add that to the sauce. If the sauce is too sour to suit you, add a little tamari, tasting as you go until you get the desired result.

Please be aware that when avocado is called for, it is to be added last unless otherwise noted. This is because avocado is a natural thickener, and if it is added too early, it may be difficult to blend the other ingredients. When added last, avocado will smoothly thicken the blended mixture, and if necessary, some extra liquid may be added to get the required texture.

Never be afraid to experiment with combinations of ingredients—you will quickly learn what works and what does not, and what suits your taste and what does not.

The following sauces are easy to prepare, and can be served with vegetables, greens, and sprouts.

ALMOND SAUCE

Yield: Approximately 1½ cups

This makes a delicious, sweetly fermented cream.

1 cup soaked almonds
2 cups *Rejuvelac* (page 38) or spring water

1. Blend all the ingredients together.
2. Put the mixture into a bowl, cover, and allow it to ferment overnight.

ALMOND-CARAWAY SEED SAUCE

Yield: Approximately 3 cups

2 cups almonds, soaked

3 cups *Rejuvelac* (page 38) or spring water

1 tablespoon caraway seeds

Juice of 2 lemons

1. Blend all the ingredients together until smooth.

2. Put the mixture in a bowl and allow it to ferment for the time suggested on page 84, depending on the liquid used.

ALMOND-SUNFLOWER SEED SAUCE

Yield: Approximately 1½ cups

½ cup soaked almonds

½ cup soaked sunflower seeds

2 cups *Rejuvelac* (page 38) or spring water

1. Blend all the ingredients together until smooth.

2. Put the mixture into a bowl, and allow it to ferment for 4 to 9 hours.

APPLE AND SUNFLOWER SAUCE

Yield: Approximately 4 cups

2 cups sunflower seed cheese (see page 40)
1 sweet apple, chopped
1 stalk celery, chopped
1 tablespoon chopped fresh dill
1 cup *Rejuvelac* (page 38) or spring water

1. Blend all the ingredients together until smooth and creamy.

2. Put the mixture in a bowl and allow it to ferment for the time suggested on page 84, depending on the liquid used.

AVOCADO DILL SAUCE

Yield: Approximately ½ cup

2 tablespoons *Rejuvelac* (page 38) or spring water
¼ cup cucumber, peeled, seeded, and chopped
1 sprig dill
¼ teaspoon lemon juice
¼ teaspoon tamari
½ ripe avocado, peeled and sliced

1. Blend all the ingredients, except the avocado, until smooth.

2. Add the avocado, and blend until smooth.

3. Put the mixture in a bowl, and allow it to ferment for the time suggested on page 84, depending on the liquid used.

AVOCADO SAUCE

Yield: Approximately 1 cup

2 tablespoons fresh lemon juice

⅓ cup *Rejuvelac* (page 38) or spring water

½ teaspoon fresh dill (optional)

1 large ripe avocado, peeled and sliced

1. Blend all the ingredients, except the avocado, together until smooth.

2. Add the avocado, and blend until smooth.

3. Put the mixture in a bowl, and allow it to ferment for the time suggested on page 84, depending on the liquid used.

Variations

More lemon juice may be added for a lighter dressing. Different herbs, such as parsley, chervil, tarragon, basil, thyme, fennel, or mint can be used to vary the taste, and to suit the dish the sauce is to be used with.

BASIC SEED OR NUT SAUCE

Yield: 3 cups

Any seeds or nuts can be used, according to your individual tastes.

2 cups seeds or nuts, ground into meal
in an electric grinder or with a hand mill

2 cups *Rejuvelac* (page 38) or spring water

1. Blend the seed or nut meal and the *Rejuvelac* or spring water until the mixture reaches a creamy consistency, resembling a milk shake.

2. Put the mixture into a bowl and allow it to ferment for the time suggested on page 84, depending on the liquid used.

Variations

To vary the basic sauce, try one of the following combinations.

- 1½ cups sunflower meal and ½ cup almond meal
- 1 cup cashew meal and 1 cup sunflower meal
- 1 cup sunflower meal and 1 cup sesame seed meal
- All sesame seed meal
- All sunflower seed meal

BEET SAUCE

Yield: Approximately 1 cup

Juice of 1½ medium beets
Juice of 1 small lemon
1 teaspoon honey

1. Blend all the ingredients together until smooth.

2. Put the mixture into a bowl and allow it to ferment for a few hours, according to your taste.

CARROT-BEET SAUCE

Yield: Approximately 2½ cups

1 cup grated carrots
1 cup sliced beets
1 tablespoon tamari
1 tablespoon kelp
1 cup *Rejuvelac* (page 38) or spring water
½ avocado, peeled and sliced

1. Blend all the ingredients, except the avocado, to the desired consistency.

2. Add the avocado, and blend again.

3. Put the mixture in a bowl, and allow it to ferment for the time suggested on page 84, depending on the liquid used.

CAULIFLOWER AND MUSHROOM SAUCE

Yield: Approximately 1½ cups

1 cup finely chopped cauliflower
1 cup finely sliced mushrooms
½ cup *Rejuvelac* (page 38) or spring water
1 tablespoon tamari
1 scallion, chopped
2 tablespoons chopped fresh parsley
Kelp and cayenne pepper to taste

1. Reserve two-thirds of the cauliflower and half the mushrooms.

2. Blend the remaining cauliflower and mushrooms with the other ingredients until smooth.

3. Put the mixture into a bowl and allow it to ferment for 2 to 3 hours.

4. Pour the sauce over the reserved vegetables, and serve as a sauced salad.

CHLOROPHYLL SAUCE

Yield: Approximately 1½ cups

1 cup spring or filtered water or *Rejuvelac*
(page 38)

4 tablespoons sunflower seed meal

2 cups sunflower greens or buckwheat lettuce

1 tablespoon kelp

1 teaspoon minced fresh parsley

½ avocado, peeled and sliced

1. Put the water or *Rejuvelac* in the blender, and gradually blend in the remaining ingredients, except the avocado.

2. Add the avocado, and blend until smooth.

3. Put the mixture in a bowl, and allow it to ferment for the time suggested on page 84, depending on the liquid used.

· CORN SAUCE

Yield: Approximately 3 cups

Kernels from 2 medium ears of corn
½ cup *Rejuvelac* (page 38) or spring water
1 bunch watercress, chopped
1 avocado, peeled and sliced

1. Blend the corn kernels with the *Rejuvelac* or spring
   water, then blend in the watercress and the avocado.
   If the sauce is too thick, add more liquid.

2. Put the mixture in a bowl, and allow it to ferment
   for the time suggested on page 84, depending on the
   liquid used.

EGGPLANT MAYONNAISE

Yield: Approximately 1 cup

The consistency of this sauce should be similar to that
of regular mayonnaise, but you may use more *Rejuvelac*
or spring water if a thinner texture is wanted.

1 cup *Rejuvelac* (page 38) or spring water
2 tablespoons sunflower seed cheese (page 40)
½ medium eggplant, peeled and diced
3 tablespoons minced parsley

1. Blend the *Rejuvelac* or spring water and the seed
   cheese, then add the eggplant and the parsley.

2. Put the mixture in a bowl, and allow it to ferment
   for the time suggested on page 84, depending on the
   liquid used.

GREEN SAUCE

Yield: Approximately 2 cups

1 cup spring or filtered water or *Rejuvelac*
(page 38)

1½ cups chopped greens, such as
Swiss chard, spinach, beet tops, celery leaves,
or whatever is in season

½ avocado, peeled and sliced

Kelp or other seasonings to taste

1. Put the water or *Rejuvelac* in the blender and add the greens a little at a time, blending until a fine consistency is reached.

2. Add the avocado, blend, and season to taste with kelp or other preferred seasoning.

3. Put the mixture in a bowl, and allow it to ferment for the time suggested on page 84, depending on the liquid used.

Variations

To change the flavor, add a few mint leaves or half a garlic clove, pressed, or one small onion, chopped, or three scallions, chopped.

GREEN HERBAL SALAD DRESSING

Yield: Approximately 2 cups

2 cups chopped mixed greens
(such as dandelion leaves, romaine lettuce,
chicory, or watercress)

⅓ cup fresh lemon juice

1 clove garlic, pressed

½ teaspoon each thyme, basil, marjoram,
and tarragon

1 teaspoon tamari

½ avocado, peeled and sliced

1. Blend all the ingredients, except the avocado, until smooth.

2. Add the avocado, and blend well.

3. Put the mixture into a bowl and allow it to ferment for a few hours, according to your taste.

GINGER SAUCE

Yield: Approximately 3 cups

This sauce is highly nutritious—it contains vitamins A, B complex, D, and E, as well as minerals—and can be used as a salad dressing, over vegetables, or as a dip.

1 cup soaked almonds

2 cups *Rejuvelac* (page 38) or spring water

2 tablespoons peeled and chopped fresh ginger

2 tablespoons lemon juice

1 avocado, peeled and sliced

1. Blend all the ingredients, except the avocado, together until smooth.

2. Add the avocado, and blend until smooth.

3. Put the mixture into a bowl, and allow it to ferment for the time suggested on page 84, depending on the liquid used.

GOLDEN SAUCE

Yield: Approximately 2 cups

½ small zucchini, chopped
½ cup *Rejuvelac* (page 38) or spring water
1 stalk celery, sliced
½ medium carrot, chopped
1 teaspoon kelp
Pinch cayenne pepper
1 cup any kind of sprouts
½ avocado, peeled and sliced

1. Blend the zucchini and the *Rejuvelac* or spring water.

2. Add the other ingredients, except the avocado, and blend until smooth.

3. Add the avocado, and blend until smooth.

4. Put the mixture in a bowl, and allow it to ferment for the time suggested on page 84, depending on the liquid used.

MUSHROOM SAUCE

Yield: Approximately 2 cups

1 cup chopped mushrooms
½ cup *Rejuvelac* (page 38) or spring water
¼ cup ground cashews
1–2 teaspoons tamari, to taste
1 teaspoon paprika

1. Blend all the ingredients together until smooth.

2. Put the mixture in a bowl, and allow it to ferment for the time suggested on page 84, depending on the liquid used.

Variation

Add 1 cup alfalfa sprouts, 1 medium tomato, sliced, or a small bunch of parsley, chopped.

PARSLEY SAUCE

Yield: Approximately 1 cup

½ cup sunflower seeds, soaked for 5 hours, drained, and allowed to sprout for one day
2 sprigs parsley
2 scallions, chopped
½ cup *Rejuvelac* (page 38) or spring water

1. Blend all the ingredients together until smooth.

2. Put the mixture in a bowl, and allow it to ferment for the time suggested on page 84, depending on the liquid used.

QUICK AND EASY VEGETABLE SAUCE

Yield: Approximately 2 cups

Almost any combination of vegetables can be used. For example, a red sauce is produced by blending tomatoes, carrots, and squash. If avocado is not available, soaked nuts or seeds, such as sunflower or sesame seeds, almonds, cashews, or pine nuts, can be substituted as a thickener.

1 cup mixed, chopped vegetables

1 cup *Rejuvelac* (page 38) or spring water

1 cup any kind of seaweed

1 avocado, peeled and sliced

1. Blend all the ingredients, except the avocado, together until smooth.

2. Add the avocado, and blend until smooth.

3. Put the mixture in a bowl, and allow it to ferment for the time suggested on page 84, depending on the liquid used.

Variations

Different herbs and spices can be used to alter the flavor of the sauce. Try 1 to 2 tablespoons chopped fresh basil, dill, cilantro, scallions, or grated ginger.

RADISH AND TOMATO SAUCE

Yield: ½ cup

2 ripe tomatoes, sliced

3 red radishes, chopped, or
½ cup radish sprouts

1 tablespoon lemon juice

1. Blend all the ingredients together until smooth.

2. Put the mixture in a bowl and allow it to ferment for a few hours, according to your taste.

SESAME AND SUNFLOWER SEED SAUCE

Yield: Approximately 3 cups

1 cup sunflower seeds

Pinch cayenne pepper

1 cup sesame seed meal

1 teaspoon tamari

2 cups *Rejuvelac* (page 38) or spring water
(use more, if necessary)

1. Soak the sunflower seeds for 5 to 6 hours, drain, and rinse.

2. Blend all the ingredients together until smooth. Add more *Rejuvelac* or spring water if a thinner sauce is wanted.

3. Put the mixture in a bowl, and allow it to ferment for the time suggested on page 84, depending on the liquid used.

SPECIAL AVOCADO MAYONNAISE

Yield: Approximately 1½ cups

Like the Eggplant Mayonnaise on page 92, the consistency of this sauce should be similar to that of regular mayonnaise, but more liquid may be added if a thinner sauce is desired.

1 small avocado, peeled and sliced

½ cup *Rejuvelac* (page 38) or spring water

1 cup cashews or pecans, soaked overnight
and ground into meal

1 tablespoon honey

1. Blend the avocado with the *Rejuvelac* or spring water.

2. Slowly blend in the nut meal, then the honey.

3. Put the mixture in a bowl, and allow it to ferment for the time suggested on page 84, depending on the liquid used.

Variation

Substitute ½ cup carrot or tomato juice for the *Rejuvelac* or spring water.

SPINACH DRESSING

Yield: Approximately 2 cups

1 avocado, peeled and sliced
½ cup *Rejuvelac* (page 38) or spring water
1 cup chopped spinach leaves
½ bunch watercress, chopped
¹/₈ teaspoon ground ginger
¹/₈ teaspoon kelp

1. Blend the avocado with the water or *Rejuvelac*.

2. Add the remaining ingredients, and blend.

3. Put the mixture in a bowl, and allow it to ferment for the time suggested on page 84, depending on the liquid used.

SPROUTED PUMPKIN SEED SAUCE

Yield: Approximately 4 cups

2 cups sprouted pumpkin seeds
1 teaspoon kelp or dulse
2 scallions, chopped
2 stalks celery, chopped
½ cup grated beets
Juice of 1 lemon
Enough *Rejuvelac* to blend

1. Blend all the ingredients together until smooth.

2. Put the mixture in a bowl, and allow it to ferment for 8 hours or overnight.

Variation

Substitute 2 cups chopped pumpkin for the sprouted pumpkin seeds, and proceed as above. Add extra *Rejuvelac* or spring water if a thinner sauce is required. This version does not need to ferment overnight, but can be served over salad or vegetables when blending is completed.

SQUASH SAUCE

Yield: Approximately 2½ cups

1 medium squash, grated

1 stalk celery, chopped

½ tomato, sliced

2 scallions, chopped

¼ cup *Rejuvelac* (page 38) or spring water

½ bell pepper, chopped

½ teaspoon your choice of seasoning

3 basil leaves

½ avocado, peeled and sliced

1. Blend all the ingredients, except the avocado, to the desired texture.

2. Add the avocado, and blend again. Add more liquid if necessary.

3. Put the mixture in a bowl, and allow it to ferment for the time suggested on page 84, depending on the liquid used.

SUNFLOWER SEED SAUCE

Yield: Approximately 2½ cups

1 cup sunflower seeds

2 cups *Rejuvelac* (page 38) or spring water

1 teaspoon tamari

4 tablespoons lemon juice

1 tablespoon honey

1 teaspoon paprika

1 tablespoon chopped fresh basil

1. Soak the sunflower seeds for 5 to 6 hours, drain, and rinse.

2. Blend the soaked seeds with the remaining ingredients until smooth.

3. Put the mixture in a bowl, and allow it to ferment for up to 5 hours.

ZUCCHINI SAUCE

Yield: Approximately 1 cup

1 small zucchini, chopped

1 tablespoon tamari

1 stalk celery, chopped

½ cup *Rejuvelac* (page 38) or spring water

4 sprigs parsley, chopped

1. Blend all the ingredients together until smooth.

2. Put the mixture in a bowl, and allow it to ferment for the time suggested on page 84, depending on the liquid used.

FRUIT SAUCES AND CREAMS

The following sauces are slightly sweeter than the others in this chapter. They should be fermented for a shorter period of time; about two to three hours is sufficient if *Rejuvelac* is used. If spring water is used, the sauce should be fermented for several more hours. This is long enough to give the sauce a flavor that is rich, but not too strong. Some recipes, such as Fruit Dressing (page 106), contain neither water nor *Rejuvelac*. These should be fermented for just a few hours, according to your own taste. These sauces can be served with fruits or fruit salads, as long as acid fruits are not used.

APPLE SAUCE

Yield: Approximately 2 cups

2 Golden Delicious apples, peeled, cored, and chopped

½ cup *Rejuvelac* (page 38) or spring water

4 figs, sliced

⅛ teaspoon cinnamon

1. Blend all the ingredients together until smooth.

2. Put the mixture in a bowl and allow it to ferment for the time suggested above, depending on the liquid used.

BANANA AND APPLE SAUCE

Yield: Approximately 3 cups

1 banana

2 apples, peeled, cored, and chopped

5 soaked dates, chopped

1 cup *Rejuvelac* (page 38) or spring water

Maple syrup to taste

1. Blend all the ingredients together until smooth.

2. Put the mixture in a bowl and allow it to ferment for the time suggested on page 103, depending on the liquid used.

CASHEW CREAM

Yield: Approximately 4 cups

1 cup soaked cashew nuts

1 cup *Rejuvelac* (page 38) or spring water

4 Golden Delicious apples, peeled, cored, and chopped

1. Blend all the ingredients together until smooth.

2. Put the mixture in a bowl and allow it to ferment for the time suggested on page 103, depending on the liquid used.

COCONUT AND APPLE SAUCE

Yield: Approximately 3 cups

2 cups chopped apples

4 tablespoons chopped or shredded coconut

1 cup soaked almonds

5 soaked dates

2 cups *Rejuvelac* (page 38) or spring water

1. Blend all the ingredients together until smooth.

2. Put the mixture in a bowl and allow it to ferment for the time suggested on page 103, depending on the liquid used.

COCONUT SAUCE

Yield: Approximately 2 cups

1 cup orange juice

1 orange, peeled and chopped

½ cup shredded coconut

1 tablespoon lemon or lime juice

½ cup *Rejuvelac* (page 38) or spring water

1. Blend all the ingredients together until smooth.

2. Put the mixture in a bowl and allow it to ferment for the time suggested on page 103, depending on the liquid used.

DATE BUTTER

Yield: Approximately ½ cup

½ cup soaked, pitted dates

½ cup *Rejuvelac* (page 38) or spring water

1. Blend all the ingredients together until smooth.

2. Put the mixture in a bowl and allow it to ferment for the time suggested on page 103, depending on the liquid used.

Variation

Use any kind of dried fruit, and soak for 2 to 4 hours before blending.

FRUIT DRESSING

Yield: Approximately 1 cup

½ cup orange juice

¼ cup pineapple juice

¼ cup lemon juice

1 avocado, peeled and cut up

1. Put the juices into the blender, add the avocado, and blend until smooth.

2. Put the mixture in a bowl and allow it to ferment for a few hours, according to taste.

MELLOW CREAM

Yield: Approximately 1 cup

1 cup chopped cantaloupe
¼ cup chopped honeydew
Juice of 1 small lime

1. Blend all the ingredients together.

2. Put the mixture in a bowl and allow it to ferment for a few hours, according to taste.

3. Serve as a sauce for melon salads.

PINEAPPLE COCONUT SAUCE

Yield: Approximately 2 cups

2 cups chopped pineapple
½ cup shredded coconut
2 tablespoons lemon or lime juice
½ cup *Rejuvelac* (page 38) or spring water
(optional)

1. Blend all the ingredients together until smooth. Add the *Rejuvelac* or spring water if a thinner sauce is desired.

2. Put the mixture in a bowl and allow it to ferment for the time suggested on page 103, depending on the liquid used.

SESAME COCONUT SAUCE

Yield: Approximately 2½ cups

1 cup shredded coconut
1 cup sprouted sesame seeds
3 tablespoons honey
2 cups *Rejuvelac* (page 38) or spring water

1. Blend all the ingredients together until smooth.

2. Put the mixture in a bowl and allow it to ferment for the time suggested on page 103, depending on the liquid used.

8

Desserts

Last, but certainly not least, blending can be used to create some unique and healthful desserts. Since fruits and vegetables are poor combinations at the same meal, it is best to wait at least one hour, and preferably two, between a vegetable-based meal and a fruit dessert. The puddings and desserts listed below can tempt any sweet tooth without presenting the health hazards that accompany commercially produced goods baked with refined sugar, flour, and oils, but they are not recommended for use more than three to four times a week (unless you are trying to gain weight). For added variety when you do have desserts, try the many fruit beverages and sauces listed in other chapters of this book.

Whether dining alone or having company, you can serve these desserts with all the pride of an accomplished cook, and with the added satisfaction that you are providing your guests with tempting treats that are as healthful as they are delicious.

BANANA COCONUT PIE

Yield: 8 servings

Crust:

1 cup finely ground almonds

1 cup black figs or dates, soaked for 1 hour

½ teaspoon ground cloves

1 cup raisins, soaked for 1 hour

Filling:

4 bananas

½ cup *Rejuvelac* (page 38) or spring water
or freshly made apple juice

1 cup grated coconut

6 dates, soaked

2 teaspoons honey

1 teaspoon pure vanilla extract

Raisins, currants, apple slices, or
shredded coconut for garnish

1. To make the pie crust, blend all the pie crust ingredients together, and press into a 9-inch pie pan. Set aside.

2. Mash two of the bananas with a fork, and put them into the blender with the *Rejuvelac* or apple juice, ½ cup of the coconut, and the dates, honey, and vanilla. Blend until smooth, and put into a bowl.

3. Slice the remaining bananas and add them and the remainder of the coconut to the blended mixture. Mix gently, but well.

4. Spread the filling mixture into the crust and refrigerate until needed.

5. The pie can be decorated just before serving with raisins or currants, apple slices, or a sprinkle of shredded coconut.

BANANA ICE CREAM WITH ALMOND CREME SAUCE

Yield: 1 cup

The amount of ice cream can be varied depending on the number of bananas used.

Ice Cream:

2 overripe bananas

Sauce:

1 cup peeled, soaked almonds
(see page 40 for instructions on peeling almonds)

2 cups *Rejuvelac* (page 38), spring water,
or water in which dried fruits were soaked

2 bananas

1 tablespoon carob powder

Raisins or honey to taste

1. To make the ice cream, peel and freeze the bananas in single layers in plastic bags, two days in advance.

2. Run the frozen bananas through the Champion juicer, using the blank juicer part rather than the screen, or process them in a food processor until mashed. It is advisable to chill the machine parts first, or the bananas will be too soft as they come through.

3. Put the banana pulp in a dish and chill in the freezer, preferably overnight.

4. To make the sauce, blend the almonds with the *Rejuvelac* or water until smooth.

5. Add the remaining ingredients and blend until creamy.

6. Refrigerate the sauce; use as a topping for banana ice cream.

Variations

Other fruits can be added to the ice cream. These can be dried, fresh, or frozen. Try berries, pineapple, figs, pitted dates, peaches, pears, or cantaloupe. If you choose dried fruits, cut them into small pieces and sprinkle on top of the ice cream, or soak them for 1 to 2 hours and put them through the Champion juicer with the bananas. If you use fresh fruits, cut them up and mix with the ice cream. Frozen fruit can be put through the juicer with the bananas.

To make chocolate ice cream, add 2 teaspoons carob powder for every five bananas used. This should be added after the ice cream has been frozen.

BANANA PUDDING

Yield: Approximately 7 cups

6 ripe bananas

½ cup freshly made apple juice

1½ cups raisins

¼ teaspoon nutmeg

1 tablespoon honey

1. Blend all the ingredients together until smooth.

2. Put the mixture in the refrigerator until chilled, and serve.

BANANA-ALMOND CREAM PIE

Yield: 8 servings

Crust:

1 cup finely ground almonds
1 cup black figs, soaked for 1 hour
1 cup raisins, soaked for 1 hour
½ teaspoon cinnamon

Filling:

2 cups almond meal
3 bananas
1 teaspoon nutmeg
½–1 cup *Rejuvelac* (page 38) or spring water
Banana slices, raisins, and
shredded coconut for garnish

1. To make the pie crust, blend all the pie crust ingredients together. Press this mixture into a 9-inch pie pan, and set aside.

2. To prepare the filling, blend the almond meal, bananas, and nutmeg. Add enough *Rejuvelac* or spring water to give the mixture a thick, pudding-like consistency.

3. Put the filling mixture into the freezer and chill until firm, between 1 and 2 hours.

4. Remove the filling from the freezer and pack into the crust. Decorate with a few banana slices, raisins, and shredded coconut, and serve.

CAROB BANANA CREAM PIE

Crust:

1 cup dates, raisins, or figs, soaked for 1 hour
(reserve the soaking water and a few fruits
for garnish)

1 cup almonds or walnuts, soaked and ground
(reserve some for garnish)

1 cup shredded coconut (reserve some for garnish)

Filling:

7 bananas, sliced (reserve a few slices for garnish)

⅓ cup carob powder

1. To make the pie crust, use some of the water in
   which the fruit was soaked to blend the fruit to a
   purée. Reserve 1 cup of the puréed fruit.

2. Mix the remainder of the puréed fruit with the
   ground nuts and the coconut until a doughy consistency is reached. Press this mixture into a 9-inch pie
   pan, and set aside.

3. To make the filling, blend the bananas with the remainder of the soaking water until smooth. Spread
   half of this mixture into the pie crust, then spread
   the reserved fruit purée over this layer.

4. Thoroughly mix the remaining half of the banana
   mixture with the carob powder and spread this mixture on top of the fruit purée.

5. Decorate the pie with the reserved banana slices,
   dates, ground nuts, and coconut.

6. Put the pie into the freezer and chill for 1 hour before serving.

FRUIT MINCE

Yield: 3½ cups

This can be eaten by itself or made into a pie, using the Banana-Almond Cream Pie crust on page 113.

1 cup raisins, soaked for 1 hour

1 teaspoon honey

1 cup pitted dates, soaked for 1 hour, then chopped

1 teaspoon cinnamon

1 cup grated apple

½ teaspoon nutmeg

½ teaspoon ground cloves

1. Blend all the ingredients together.

2. If the resulting mixture is too rich for your taste, it can be lightened by stirring in extra grated fruit (such as plums, nectarines, peaches, or fresh pineapple, as available and as preferred.) For a thinner mince, some of the additional fruit may be blended before it is mixed in.

MIXED FRUIT PIE

Any kind of nuts, seeds, or dried fruits may be used for this pie, but they must be soaked first. Filberts and peeled almonds should be soaked for 24 hours; sunflower seeds should be soaked for 5 to 6 hours; and pine nuts (pignoli) should be soaked for 4 hours. Dried fruit should be soaked for 3 to 6 hours.

Crust:

1 cup mixed nuts and seeds, such as almonds, filberts, or sunflower seeds.

2 cups soaked dried fruit, such as figs, dates, raisins, or prunes

Filling:

4 bananas

15 dates, chopped

1 cup shredded coconut or
¼ cup carob powder (optional)

Topping:

⅔ cup pine nuts

⅓ cup dates

½–1 cup *Rejuvelac* (page 38) or spring water

1. To make the pie crust, blend all the pie crust ingredients together. Spread the mixture into a 9-inch pie pan, and set aside.

2. To make the filling, blend the bananas and the dates until smooth. Add the coconut or carob powder if desired. Pour this mixture into the pie crust.

3. To make the topping, blend the pine nuts and dates

together, adding just enough *Rejuvelac* or spring water
to give the mixture a smooth texture. Spread on top
of the completed pie.

Variation

Instead of bananas and dates, use 1 cup chopped apples and 2 cups prunes, or 3 cups peeled fresh or dried
fruit, for the topping. Blend until smooth, and proceed
as above.

PAPAYA SHERBET

Yield: Approximately 1½ cups

½ small ripe papaya, peeled and cut up
1 slice fresh pineapple, chopped
½ ripe banana, sliced
½ teaspoon pure vanilla extract
Juice of 1 orange
1 teaspoon honey

1. Blend the papaya until smooth.

2. Put the blended papaya into a bowl and mix in the
   other ingredients.

3. Put the mixture into a freezer tray, and freeze until
   almost set, about 2 to 3 hours.

4. Remove the mixture from the freezer and whip in the
   blender until smooth.

5. Return the sherbet to the freezer for 2 to 3 more
   hours, and serve.

PEACH ICE CREAM

Yield: Approximately 6 cups

5 very ripe bananas
2 large ripe peaches, chopped

1. Blend the bananas until smooth.

2. Turn the banana mixture into a dish and add the peach chunks.

3. Freeze the mixture for at least 4 hours before serving.

Variation

1 cup of blueberries, strawberries, or chopped mango or papaya can be added to the mixture.

PEAR PUDDING—VARIATION #1

Yield: Approximately 4 cups

An equal amount of other seasonal fruits may be added to the pears in this and the following recipe. Try bananas, papayas, persimmons, pineapples, honeydew, or cantaloupe.

3 cups peeled, cored, and diced pears
$1/3$ cup soaked raisins
1 cup chopped pineapple
2 cups diced papaya
¼ cup soaked currants and
¼ teaspoon cinnamon for garnish

1. Blend all the ingredients together until smooth.

2. Garnish with the currants and cinnamon.

PEAR PUDDING—VARIATION #2

Yield: Approximately 4 cups

5 soaked dried figs

3 cups peeled, cored, and diced fresh pears

3 cups peeled and diced ripe persimmons

¼ cup soaked currants and
¼ teaspoon cinnamon for garnish

1. Blend all the ingredients together until smooth.

2. Garnish with the currants and cinnamon.

PERSIMMON PUDDING

Yield: Approximately 5 cups

3 ripe bananas, sliced

1 tablespoon honey

4 ripe persimmons, peeled and sliced

1 teaspoon pure vanilla extract

1. Blend all the ingredients together.

2. Place the mixture in the freezer, chill until smooth, and serve.

Conclusion

I hope and pray that you now have an understanding of what you will need to do in order to change your life in a positive way. This book has been carefully arranged and thought out in order to make blending foods simpler than ever for you to understand. It is so vital for us to realize, especially at this time, the importance of being self-sufficient and of eating for nourishment, rather than just for the sake of eating. I hope that you will recognize that the body always has been and always will be a self-healer. It cannot fail if you work with nature, rather than against it.

There is an incredible need for all of us to become interested in the tools of nature. When we use blended live foods in a balanced diet, we not only balance our own lives, but we become able to balance our planet. Through your own efforts, you will gain confidence that your body's capabilities will provide the needed results, enabling you to accomplish what you want to accomplish in your lifetime. As you connect with nature, you are connecting with your higher self.

Therefore, you will be able to share your good health with your family and friends, and will be able to really help them with their needs if they are ready.

There are many of us trying to right the conditions of the world. It is time for people to realize that all aspects of health—physical, mental, and emotional—must be taken into consideration before any of the problems that are so difficult to handle can be erased. The government and other institutions cannot possibly help at this time unless every one of us becomes an example of good health. We must become examples not only for our families, but for the whole world.

I hope you will consider the information in this book as a way of opening doors for yourself and for your loved ones.

With loving heart,

Dr. Ann Wigmore

Appendices

To maintain optimum health and energy, it is essential that we take in adequate amounts of nutrients. A knowledge of what we need and how those needs can be met is very important. Since all of the foods eaten in the living foods lifestyle are uncooked, their full vitamin and mineral values are available to the body.

The first chart in this section shows the recommended daily intake of protein and calories, broken down according to age. This is followed by a chart entitled *Essential Vitamins and Minerals—and What They Do*. This chart shows the amount of each nutrient according to the recommended daily allowance (RDA) established by the U.S. government. The values given are for adult males; those for adult females are slightly lower. Alongside the RDAs, you will find the estimated values of each nutrient supplied by the living foods lifestyle. The living foods lifestyle provides an adult with more than two times the RDA for almost every nutrient.

Following the vitamin and mineral chart, I have included a handy *Composition of Foods* chart for easy reference to many of the foods commonly eaten in the living foods lifestyle.

With the information in these charts, you can easily determine if you are taking in all that you need to meet your body's requirements and to keep your energy level at its peak. If you are below par, a study of these charts will enable you to make any necessary adjustments to insure that you have a balanced diet of maximum benefit that suits your individual lifestyle.

DAILY PROTEIN AND CALORIE CHARTS

INFANTS			
Age	**Weight** (pounds)	**Protein** (g/day)	**Calories*** (per day)
Newborn–6 mos.	13	13	650
6 mos.–1 year	20	14	850

*In the range of light to moderate activity, the coefficient of variation is ±20%.

CHILDREN			
Age (years)	**Weight** (pounds)	**Protein** (grams)	**Calories**
1–3	29	16	1300
4–6	44	24	1800
7–10	62	28	2000

MALES			
Age (years)	**Weight** (pounds)	**Protein** (grams)	**Calories**
11–14	99	45	2500
15–18	145	59	3000
19–24	160	58	2900
25–50	174	63	2900
51+	170	63	2300

FEMALES			
Age (years)	**Weight** (pounds)	**Protein** (grams)	**Calories**
11–14	101	46	2200
15–18	120	44	2200
19–24	128	46	2200
25–50	138	50	2200
51+	143	50	1900

During pregnancy, add 30 grams of protein and 300 calories to the above totals. While lactating, add 20 grams of protein and 500 calories to the above totals.

ESSENTIAL VITAMINS AND MINERALS CHART— AND WHAT THEY DO

Vitamins	Food Sources	Function in Body	RDA (adult)*	Estimated Wigmore Diet Value**
A (carotene)	alfalfa sprouts, kale, apricots, carrots, dandelion greens, leafy greens, orange & yellow vegetables, tomatoes, peaches, wheatgrass	Aids normal growth, reproduction, and development. Aids skin, teeth, mucous membranes, and eyesight. Maintains resistance to infection	5000 I.U	30,000–50,000 I.U.

Vitamins	Food Sources	Function in Body	RDA (adult)*	Estimated Wigmore Diet Value**
B₁ (thiamine)	alfalfa sprouts, bean sprouts, citrus fruits, grain sprouts, leafy greens, nuts, pine nuts, sunflower seeds, vegetables	Aids assimilation of starches and sugars; builds appetite and energy. Aids digestion, the heart, and the liver.	1.2–2.0 mg.	2.1–4.7 mg.
B₂ (riboflavin)	alfalfa sprouts, almonds, bananas, citrus fruits, kelp, leafy greens, mushrooms, tomatoes, soy sprouts, sprouted beans and grains	Improves resistance to disease. Aids normal growth and development. Improves skin and eyesight.	1.6–2.6 mg.	2.7–3.97 mg.
B₁₂	bean sprouts, dulse, wheatgrass	Prevents nerve cell degeneration. Aids formation of red blood cells.	3–5 mcg.	5 mcg.
Niacin (a B vitamin)	alfalfa sprouts, kelp, leafy greens, pine nuts, sesame seeds, sprouted beans and grains, sunflower seeds, tomatoes	Aids mental health and nervous system. Helps maintain appetite and adrenal health.	12–20 mg.	26–32.5 mg.
C (ascorbic acid)	cherries, fruits, kale, leafy greens, melons, oranges and other citrus fruits, parsley, red peppers, sprouts, tomatoes, wheatgrass	Aids growth and development. Maintains tissues, joints, ligaments, teeth, and gums. Promotes healing and resistance to infection.	75–100 mg.	300–418.8 mg.
D	almonds, coconuts, sunflower seeds, sunlight	Promotes normal formation of strong bones and teeth.	400 I.U.	400 I.U.

Vitamins	Food Sources	Function in Body	RDA (adult)*	Estimated Wigmore Diet Value**
E	beets, celery, leafy greens, nuts and seeds, oils, sprouted grains, wheatgrass	Aids reproduction, the heart, and the utilization of fatty acids.	10–30 mg.	20–45 mg.
K	alfalfa sprouts, leafy greens, sprouted grains	Aids blood coagulation. Decreases risk of hemorrhage in pregnancy.	—	—
Minerals				
Calcium	almonds, dandelion greens, dulse, filberts, kale, kelp, leafy greens, nuts, parsley, sesame seeds and sprouts, sprouts, watercress, wheatgrass	Builds healthy bones and teeth. Helps blood clot. Regulates heartbeat and mineral balance.	800 mg.	1500–2072 mg.
Chlorine	avocados, celery, kale, kelp, lettuce, radishes, red cabbage, spinach, tomatoes	Aids digestion and elimination. Sustains normal heart activity.	trace	trace
Iodine	dulse, kelp, leafy greens, wheatgrass	Stimulates thyroid gland, which regulates rate of digestion. Important for growth and development.	—	.7 mg.
Iron	bean sprouts, dulse, fruits (dried and fresh), kelp, leafy greens, lentil sprouts, nuts, seeds	Helps form hemoglobin and myoglobin. Aids oxygen transport to cells and prevents anemia.	10 mg.	40–72.6 mg.

Minerals	Food Sources	Function in Body	RDA (adult)*	Estimated Wigmore Diet Value**
Phosphorus	bean sprouts, dulse, fruits, kelp, nuts, pumpkin and squash seeds, sesame seeds and sprouts, sprouted grains, sunflower seeds and sprouts, vegetables, wheatgrass	Builds and maintains bones, teeth, hair, and nervous tissue. Assists cells in absorbing fats and carbohydrates.	800 mg.	2500–4186 mg.
Potassium	bananas, bean sprouts, cabbage, dried fruits, dulse, fruits, leafy greens, nuts, wheatgrass	Maintains mineral balance and weight. Tones muscles. Aids disposition, promotes beauty.	—	14,452 mg.
Sodium	asparagus, celery, cucumbers, dulse, kelp, olives, sesame seeds and sprouts, sprouts, watercress	Aids digestion, speeds elimination of carbon dioxide, and regulates body fluids and heart action.	—	200–362.3 mg.

Abbreviations used in the above table:

I.U. — *International Units*
mg. — *milligrams*
mcg. — *micrograms*

Sources:

*RDAs: The figures used are adapted from the RDAs established for adult males by the U.S. Food and Drug Administration in 1980.

**Estimated nutritional content of the Ann Wigmore diet (for one person, for one day) is based on USDA *Composition of Foods Handbook No. 8.*

Composition of Foods Chart
Values for edible parts of foods.

FRUIT/raw	Amount	Grams	WATER %	FOOD ENERGY Cal.	PROTEIN g	FAT g	CARBOHYDRATE g
Apple, unpeeled w/o core and stem (3¼" diam.); appr. 2 per lb.	1 Apple	230	84.4	123	.4	1.3	30.7
Apricot, whole w/o pits; 12 per lb.	3 Apricots	114	85.3	55	1.1	.2	13.7
Avocado, cubes (½")	1 cup	150	74.0	251	3.2	24.6	9.5
Banana, w/o skin (11" long, 2" diam.)	1 Banana	365	66.4	313	2.9	1.1	82.0
Blackberries	1 cup	144	84.5	84	1.7	1.3	18.6
Blueberries	1 cup	145	83.2	90	1.0	.7	22.2
Cantaloupe, whole (cubed or diced pieces, melon balls); appr. 20 per cup	1 cup	160	91.2	48	1.4	.2	12.0
Cherries, w/o pits and stems	1 cup	145	80.4	102	1.9	.4	25.2
Dates, w/o pits	10 Dates	80	22.5	219	1.8	.4	58.3
Fig, (2½" diam.); appr. 7 per lb.	1 Fig	65	77.5	52	.8	.2	13.2
Grapefruit, whole w/o peel, seeds, and core (3½" diam.)	1 Grapefruit	400	88.4	80	1.0	.2	20.8
Grapes, seedless	1 cup	160	81.4	107	1.0	.5	27.7
Honeydew, whole w/o seed and skin (cubed or diced pcs., mellon balls); appr. 20 per cup	1 cup	170	90.6	56	1.4	.5	13.1
Lemon, fresh juice	1 tbsp.	15.2	91.0	4	.1	trace	1.2
Lemon, peel, grated	1 tbsp.	6.0	81.6	—	.1	trace	1.0
Mango, whole w/o seed and skin; diced or sliced	1 cup	165	81.7	109	1.2	.7	27.7
Nectarine, w/o pits (2½" diam.)	1 Nectarine	150	81.8	88	.8	—	23.6
Orange, cup-up (bite-size pcs.)	1 cup	165	86.0	81	1.7	.3	20.1
Papaya, cubed	1 cup	140	88.7	55	.8	.1	14.0
Peach, whole, peeled w/o skin and pits (2½" diam.); appr. 4 per lb.	1 Peach	115	89.1	38	.6	.1	9.7
Pear, sliced or cubed	1 cup	165	83.2	101	1.2	.7	25.2
Pineapple, diced	1 cup	155	85.3	81	.6	.3	21.2
Plum, pitted, halves	1 cup	170	81.1	112	.9	—	30.3
Prune, pitted, halves	1 cup	165	78.7	124	1.5	.3	32.5
Prune, dried, softened, w/o pits	1 cup	180	28.0	459	308	1.1	121.3
Raisins, seedless, whole	1 cup	145	18.0	419	3.6	.3	112.2
Raspberries, black	1 cup	134	80.8	98	2.0	1.9	21.0

CALCIUM	PHOSPHORUS	IRON	SODIUM	POTASSIUM	VITAMIN A	THIAMIN	RIBOFLAVIN	NIACIN	ASCORBIC ACID
mg	mg	mg	mg	mg	mg	mg	mg	mg	mg
15	21	.6	2	233	190	.06	.04	.2	8
18	25	.5	1	301	2890	.03	.04	.6	11
15	63	.9	6	906	440	.17	.3	2.4	21
18	79	1.8	13	1012	—	.16	.11	1.6	37
46	27	1.3	1	245	290	.04	.06	.6	30
22	19	1.5	1	117	150	.04	.09	.7	20
22	26	.6	19	402	5440	.06	.05	1.0	53
32	28	.6	3	277	160	.07	.09	.6	15
47	50	2.4	1	518	40	.07	.08	1.8	0
23	14	.4	1	126	50	.04	.03	.3	1
31	31	.8	2	265	160	.08	.04	.4	74
19	32	.6	5	277	160	.08	.05	.5	6
24	27	.7	20	427	70	.07	.05	1.0	39
1	2	trace	trace	21	trace	trace	trace	trace	7
8	1	trace	trace	10	trace	trace	trace	trace	8
17	21	.7	12	312	7920	.08	.08	1.8	58
6	33	.7	8	406	2280	—	—	—	18
68	33	.7	2	330	330	.17	.07	.7	83
28	22	.4	4	328	2450	.06	.06	.4	78
9	19	.5	1	202	1330	.02	.05	1.0	7
13	18	.5	3	215	30	.03	.07	.2	7
26	12	.8	2	226	110	.14	.05	.3	26
31	29	.9	3	508	510	.14	.05	.9	—
20	30	.8	2	281	500	.05	.05	.8	7
92	142	7.0	14	1249	2880	.16	.31	2.9	5
90	146	5.1	39	1106	30	.16	.12	.7	1
40	29	1.2	1	267	trace	.04	.12	1.2	24

			WATER	FOOD ENERGY	PROTEIN	FAT	CARBOHYDRATE
FRUITS/raw (continued)	Amount	Grams	%	Cal.	g	g	g
Raspberries, red	1 cup	123	84.2	70	1.5	.6	16.7
Strawberries	1 cup	149	89.9	55	1.0	.7	12.5
Tangerine, whole w/o peel and seeds (sections w/o membranes)	1 cup	195	87.0	90	1.6	.4	22.6
Watermelon, diced pieces	1 cup	160	92.6	42	.8	.3	10.2
GRAINS/raw							
Barley, pearled, light	½ cup	100	11.1	349	8.2	1.0	78.8
Buckwheat, whole grain	½ cup	100	11.0	335	11.7	2.4	72.9
Rice, brown	½ cup	100	12.0	360	7.5	1.9	77.4
Wheat, whole, hard red winter	½ cup	100	12.5	330	12.3	1.8	71.7
Wheat, whole, soft red winter	½ cup	100	14.0	326	10.2	2.0	72.1
Wheat, bran (crude comm'l milled)	½ cup	100	11.5	213	16.0	4.6	61.9
Wheat, germ (crude comm'l milled)	½ cup	100	11.5	365	26.6	10.9	46.7
NUTS and SEEDS/raw							
Almonds, shelled, whole	1 cup	142	4.7	849	26.4	77.0	27.7
Brazil Nuts, shelled	1 cup	140	4.6	916	20.0	93.7	15.5
Chestnuts, shelled	1 cup	160	52.5	310	4.6	2.4	67.4
Coconut Meat, shredded or grated	1 cup	80	50.9	277	2.6	28.2	7.5
Coconut Water, liquid from coconut	1 cup	240	94.2	53	.7	.5	11.3
Filberts (hazelnuts), shelled, whole	1 cup	135	5.8	856	17.0	84.2	22.5
Pecans, shelled	1 cup	108	3.4	742	9.9	76.9	15.8
Pine Nuts, shelled	1 cup	28	3.1	180	3.7	17.2	5.8
Pistachios, shelled	1 lb.	454	5.3	2694	87.5	243.6	86.2
Pumpkin Seeds, hulled	1 cup	140	4.4	774	40.6	65.4	21.0
Sesame Seeds, whole	1 cup	100	5.4	563	18.6	49.1	21.6
Sesame Seeds, hulled	1½ cups	100	5.5	582	18.2	53.4	17.6
Sunflower Seeds, hulled	1 cup	145	4.8	812	34.8	68.6	28.9
Walnuts, black, shelled	1 cup	125	3.1	785	25.6	74.1	18.5
LEGUMES/raw							
Beans, dried, lima	1 cup	190	10.3	658	38.8	3.0	121.6
Beans, dried, mung	1 cup	210	10.7	714	50.8	2.7	126.6
Beans, dried, navy	1 cup	205	10.9	697	45.7	3.3	125.7
Beans, dried, pinto	1 cup	190	8.3	663	43.5	2.3	121.0
Peas, green, dried seeds (whole)	1 cup	200	11.7	680	48.2	2.6	120.6

CALCIUM	PHOSPHORUS	IRON	SODIUM	POTASSIUM	VITAMIN A	THIAMIN	RIBOFLAVIN	NIACIN	ASCORBIC ACID
mg	mg	mg	mg	mg	mg	mg	mg	mg	mg
27	27	1.1	1	207	160	.04	.11	1.1	31
31	31	1.5	1	244	90	.04	.1	.9	88
78	35	.8	4	246	820	.12	.04	.2	60
11	16	.8	2	160	940	.05	.05	.3	11
16	189	2.0	3	160	0	.12	.05	3.1	0
114	282	3.1	—	448	0	.6	—	4.4	0
32	221	1.6	9	214	0	.34	.05	4.7	0
46	354	3.4	3	370	0	.52	.12	4.3	0
42	400	3.5	3	376	0	.43	.11	3.6	0
119	1276	14.9	9	1121	0	.72	.35	21	0
72	1118	9.4	3	827	0	2.01	.68	4.2	0
332	716	6.7	6	1098	0	.34	1.31	5.0	trace
260	970	4.8	1	1001	trace	1.34	.17	2.2	—
43	141	2.7	10	726	—	.35	.35	1.0	—
10	76	1.4	18	205	0	.04	.02	.4	2
48	31	.7	60	353	0	trace	trace	1.9	5
282	455	4.6	3	950	—	.62	—	1.2	trace
79	312	2.6	trace	651	140	.93	.14	1.0	2
3	171	1.5	—	—	10	.36	.07	1.3	trace
594	2268	33.1	—	4409	1040	3.04	—	6.4	0
71	1602	15.7	—	—	100	.34	.27	3.4	0
1160	616	10.5	60	725	30	.98	.24	5.4	0
110	592	2.4	—	—	—	.18	.13	5.5	0
174	1214	10.3	44	1334	70	2.84	.33	7.8	0
trace	713	7.5	4	575	380	.28	.14	.9	—
137	732	14.8	8	2905	trace	.91	.32	3.6	—
248	714	16.2	13	2159	170	.8	.44	5.5	—
295	871	16.0	39	2452	0	1.33	.45	4.9	—
257	868	12.2	19	1870	—	1.6	.4	4.2	—
128	680	10.2	70	2010	240	1.48	.58	6.0	—

	Amount	Grams	WATER %	FOOD ENERGY Cal.	PROTEIN g	FAT g	CARBOHYDRATE g
LEGUMES/raw (continued)							
Lentils, dried seeds (whole)	1 cup	190	11.1	646	46.9	2.1	114.2
Soybeans, dried seeds (whole)	1 cup	210	10.0	846	71.6	37.2	70.4
Soybean Curd (tofu)	1 lb.	454	84.8	327	35.4	19.1	10.9
VEGETABLES/raw							
Asparagus, spears, green	1 cup	135	91.7	35	3.4	.3	6.8
Black-eyed Peas, young pods w/seeds	1 cup	100	86.0	44	3.3	.3	9.5
Broccoli, stalks	1 lb.	454	89.1	145	16.3	1.4	26.8
Brussels Sprouts	1 lb.	454	85.2	204	22.2	1.8	37.6
Cabbage, ground, green	1 cup	150	92.4	36	2.0	.3	8.1
Cabbage, shredded, red	1 cup	90	90.2	28	1.8	.2	6.2
Cabbage, shredded, savoy	1 cup	70	92.0	17	1.7	.1	3.2
Cabbage, bok choy	1 cup	70	94.3	11	1.1	.1	2.0
Carrots, grated	1 cup	110	88.2	46	1.2	.2	10.7
Cauliflower, chopped	1 cup	115	91.0	31	3.1	.2	6.0
Celery, stalk, chopped	1 cup	120	94.1	20	1.1	.1	4.7
Collards, leaves with stems	1 lb.	454	86.9	181	16.3	3.2	32.7
Corn, sweet (white, yellow) husked	1 lb.	454	72.7	240	8.7	2.5	55.1
Cucumbers, not pared, sliced, w/o ends	1 cup	105	95.1	16	.9	.1	3.6
Endive	1 cup	50	93.1	10	.9	.1	2.1
Jerusalem Artichoke	1 cup	100	79.8	114	2.3	.1	16.7
Kale, leaves w/o stems	1 lb.	454	82.7	240	27.2	3.6	40.8
Lettuce, chopped or shredded, Boston	1 cup	55	95.1	8	.7	.1	1.4
Lettuce, cos or romaine	1 cup	55	94.0	10	.7	.2	1.9
Lettuce iceberg	1 cup	55	95.5	7	.5	.1	1.6
Mushrooms, chopped	1 cup	70	90.4	20	1.9	.2	3.1
Onions, chopped	1 cup	170	89.1	65	2.6	.2	14.8
Parsley, chopped	1 cup	60	85.1	26	2.2	.4	5.1
Parsnips, diced	1 cup	155	82.2	102	2.3	.8	23.1
Peas, green	1 cup	145	78.0	122	9.1	.6	20.9
Potatoes, w/o skin, chopped	1 cup	150	79.8	345	9.5	.5	77.6
Radishes, sliced	1 cup	115	94.5	20	1.2	.1	4.1
Seaweed, dulse	1 cup	100	16.6	—	—	3.2	—
Seaweed, kelp	1 cup	100	21.7	—	—	1.1	—

CALCIUM	PHOSPHORUS	IRON	SODIUM	POTASSIUM	VITAMIN A	THIAMIN	RIBOFLAVIN	NIACIN	ASCORBIC ACID
mg	mg	mg	mg	mg	mg	mg	mg	mg	mg
150	716	12.9	57	1501	110	.70	.42	3.8	—
475	1163	17.6	11	3522	170	2.31	.65	4.6	—
581	572	8.6	32	191	0	.27	.14	.5	0
30	84	1.4	3	375	1220	.24	.27	2.0	45
65	65	1.0	4	215	1600	.15	.14	1.2	33
467	354	5.0	68	1733	11340	.45	1.04	4.1	513
163	363	6.8	64	1769	2490	.45	.73	4.1	463
74	44	.6	30	350	200	.08	.08	.5	71
38	32	.7	23	241	40	.08	.05	.4	55
47	38	.6	15	188	140	.04	.06	.2	39
116	31	.6	18	214	2170	.04	.07	.6	18
41	40	.8	52	375	12,100	.07	.06	.7	9
29	64	1.3	15	339	70	.13	.12	.8	90
47	34	.4	151	409	320	.04	.04	.4	11
921	286	4.5	195	1819	29,480	.91	1.41	7.7	417
7	277	1.7	trace	699	1,000	.37	.3	4.2	30
26	28	1.2	6	168	260	.03	.04	.2	12
41	27	.9	7	147	1650	.04	.07	.3	5
14	78	3.4	—	—	20	.2	.06	1.3	4
1129	422	12.2	340	1715	45,360	.73	1.18	9.5	844
19	14	1.1	5	145	530	.03	.03	.2	4
37	14	.8	5	145	1050	.03	.04	.2	10
11	12	.3	5	96	180	.03	.03	.2	3
4	81	.6	11	290	trace	.07	.32	2.9	2
46	61	.9	17	267	70	.05	.07	.3	17
122	38	3.7	27	436	5100	.07	.16	7.0	103
70	96	.9	12	587	50	.11	.12	.2	16
38	168	2.8	3	458	930	.51	.2	4.2	39
32	240	2.7	14	1846	trace	.45	.18	6.8	91
35	36	1.2	21	370	10	.03	.03	.3	30
296	267	—	2085	8060	—	—	—	—	—
1093	240	—	3007	5273	—	—	—	—	—

VEGETABLES/raw continued	Amount	Grams	WATER %	FOOD ENERGY Cal.	PROTEIN g	FAT g	CARBOHYDRATE g
Spinach, chopped	1 cup	55	90.7	14	1.8	.2	2.4
Sweet Potatoes, (5"L x 2" D)	1 Potato	180	74.0	132	2.3	.9	29.2
Swiss Chard	1 lb.	454	91.1	113	10.9	1.4	20.9
Tomatoes, not peeled, w/o cores and stem ends (appr. 3" diam.)	1 Tomato	135	93.5	27	1.4	.2	5.8
Turnips, cubed	1 cup	155	93.6	36	1.2	.3	7.6
Turnip Greens	1 cup	145	93.2	29	3.2	.3	5.2
Watercress	1 cup	35	93.3	7	.8	.1	1.1
Zucchini, cubed	1 cup	130	94.6	22	1.6	.1	4.7

CALCIUM	PHOSPHORUS	IRON	SODIUM	POTASSIUM	VITAMIN A	THIAMIN	RIBOFLAVIN	NIACIN	ASCORBIC ACID
mg	mg	mg	mg	mg	mg	mg	mg	mg	mg
51	28	1.7	39	259	4460	.06	.11	.8	28
41	61	.9	13	315	11,920	.13	.08	.8	30
399	177	14.5	667	2495	29,480	.27	.77	2.3	145
16	33	6.0	4	300	1110	.07	.05	.9	28
54	37	.6	53	291	trace	.06	.08	.5	34
267	54	1.6	—	—	9140	.22	.35	.9	100
53	19	.6	18	99	1720	.03	.06	.3	28
36	38	.5	1	263	420	.07	.12	1.3	25

Metric Conversion

Conversion Table		
LIQUID **When You Know**	**Multiply By**	**To Determine**
teaspoons	5.0	milliliters
tablespoons	15.0	milliliters
fluid ounces	30.0	milliliters
cups	0.24	liters
pints	0.47	liters
quarts	0.95	liters
WEIGHT **When You Know**	**Multiply By**	**To Determine**
ounces	28.0	grams
pounds	0.45	kilograms

Common Liquid Conversions

Measurements	=	Liters
1/4 cup	=	0.06
1/2 cup	=	0.12
3/4 cup	=	0.18
1 cup	=	0.24
1 1/4 cups	=	0.30
1 1/2 cups	=	0.36
2 cups	=	0.48
2 1/2 cups	=	0.60
3 cups	=	0.72
3 1/2 cups	=	0.84
4 cups	=	0.96
4 1/2 cups	=	1.08
5 cups	=	1.20
5 1/2 cups	=	1.32

Measurement	=	Milliliters
1/4 teaspoon	=	1.25
1/2 teaspoon	=	2.50
3/4 teaspoon	=	3.75
1 teaspoon	=	5.00
1 1/4 teaspoons	=	6.25
1 1/2 teaspoons	=	7.50
1 3/4 teaspoons	=	8.75
2 teaspoons	=	10.0
1 tablespoon	=	15.0
2 tablespoons	=	30.0

Index